BUILDING A SUCCESSFUL PAIN MANAGEMENT PRACTICE

The Keys To
Effective Strategy Formation
And Marketing

LINDA M. VAN HORN, M.B.A.

©1999 by Linda M. Van Horn, M.B.A.

All rights reserved. Except for appropriate use in critical reviews or works of scholarship, the reproduction or use of this work in any form or by any electronic, mechanical, or other means now known or hereafter invented, including photocopying and recording, and in any information storage and retrieval system, is forbidden without written permission of the author.

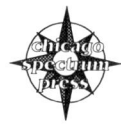

CHICAGO SPECTRUM PRESS
4824 BROWNSBORO CENTER ARCADE
LOUISVILLE, KY 40207
1-800-594-5190

Printed in the U.S.A.

10 9 8 7 6 5 4 3 2 1

ISBN: 1-886094-95-0

TABLE OF CONTENTS

INTRODUCTION 7

BOOK I: AN EFFECTIVE STRATEGIC PLAN
An Effective Strategic Plan 10
Chapter 1
Mission Statement 13
Chapter 2
Target Markets 16
Chapter 3
Competitive Analysis 22
Chapter 4
SWOT 24
Strengths 25
Weaknesses 26
Opportunities 26
Threats 27
Chapter 5
Goals of the Practice 28

BOOK II: THE KEYS TO SUCCESSFUL MARKETING
The Keys to Successful Marketing 32
Chapter 1
Needs Assessment 33
Chapter 2
Market Research 36
Satisfaction Surveys 38
Chapter 3
Creating the "Want" for Your Practice 47

Chapter 4
Service Development 49

Chapter 5
Pricing — Creating a Fee Schedule 53
Identify Every Procedure 54
Medicare Part B Fee Schedule 54
ASA Relative Value.. 57
Reimbursement Information 58
Analyze the Data 58
   FIGURE 1: ASA Relative Value Method (partial list) 60
   FIGURE 2: Cost Plus Pricing (Partial List) 63
Finalize Fee Schedule... 64
   FIGURE 3: Marketplace Average Method (partial list) 66
   FIGURE 4: Analysis Of All Methods 68

Chapter 6
Practice Name, Image, and Goodwill 70
Naming the Practice 71
The Logo Design and Color Choice 72
The Position Statement 73

Chapter 7
Choosing a Legal Entity 75
Sole Proprietorship 75
Partnership 76
Limited Liability Partnership 76
C Corporation 76
Sub-Chapter S Corporation 78
Non-Profit Organizations 78
Limited Liability Company 79
Steps to Set Up a Sub-Chapter S Corporation 79

Chapter 8
Advertising and Selling 80

Chapter 9
Timing and Packaging... 83

Chapter 10
Marketing Tools 86
Announcement 87
Business Card 90
Appointment Cards 90
Reminder Postcards 91
Rolodex® Cards 93
Brochures 94
Introduction Letters 97
Educational Packages 97
Newsletters 100

Chapter 11
Marketing Ideas 101
Direct Mail 101
Directories 103
Promotional Items 105
Professional Societies 107
Presentations to Target Markets 108
New Physicians 110
Casual Conversations and The Doctors' Lounge 112
Marketing Office Visits 112
Outgoing Referrals 115
  Federal Anti-Kickback Statute 115
  Ethics and Patients Referral Act (STARK) 116
Seasonal or Occasional Correspondence 119

Chapter 12
Media 120
Newspapers and Newsletters 122
Billboards 123
Magazines 123
Radio 124
Television (Regular and Cable) 125
Internet 126

Chapter 13
Public Relations 128
Press Releases 129
Published Articles 131
Civic Activities 132
Radio and Television Appearances 132
Chapter 14
Test Marketing 134
Chapter 15
Creating an Effective Marketing Plan 138

Postscript 150
References 151
Index 153

INTRODUCTION

*"Efficiency is doing things right.
Effectiveness is doing the right things."*
–Zig Ziglar

"Four steps to achievement: plan purposefully, prepare prayerfully, proceed positively, pursue persistently."
–William A. Ward

    The business of medicine has changed substantially over the past 10 years, and it continues to evolve. Decreasing reimbursement, increasing costs, and competition pressure physicians' practices. Healthcare, once controlled by physicians and hospitals, is now driven by multiple market forces, including managed care and government regulations. It is now more important than ever that a medical practice operate as a cost-effective and competitive business.

    Physicians, employers, and managed care executives are all disappointed with managed care's struggle to manage disease and control cost. More and more physicians and practice managers realize that creative solutions and sound business judgement are required to survive.

Current trends such as decreases in inpatient surgeries, increases in outpatient surgeries, and decreasing reimbursement have squeezed anesthesiologists' income. Many anesthesiologists have expanded or are in the process of expanding their practices to include pain management. Recognizing these trends, I have written **Building a Successful Pain Management Practice: The Keys to Strategy Formation and Marketing**.

Creating a pain management practice is dramatically different from an operating room-based practice. In the operating room, anesthesiologists perform the cases that are scheduled by the surgeons. But in pain management, they must create referrals. They must build their own practice.

Building a successful pain management practice takes time and hard work, but it is obtainable by any competent physician who is willing to plan for success. To build a successful pain management practice, you do not need a business degree, but you do need to be business-oriented and forward thinking. There is an old saying: "Failing to plan is planning to fail."

This book contains the basic business knowledge about strategy formation and marketing that is needed to create a successful pain management practice. In order to successfully market your practice you will need to commit to the preparation of two fundamental plans: *The Strategic Plan* and *The Marketing Plan*. Once these plans are developed, you need to commit to implementing the plans. This book contains the information needed to write these two plans in chronological order to help you plan, organize, and market your practice. If you are interested in finding out more about these topics, there is a list of reference books at the end of this book.

AN EFFECTIVE STRATEGIC PLAN

BOOK I
An Effective Strategic Plan

"Cheshire Puss," she began . . . "would you please tell me which way I ought to go from here?"
"That depends on the here you want to get to," said the cat.
–Lewis Carroll

"Nothing is more difficult, and therefore more precious, than the ability to decide."
–Napoleon Bonaparte

An effective strategic plan is a straightforward document that defines the practice that you want to develop. No two practices will have the same strategic plan. Strategy formation involves the assessment of your practice's capabilities and environmental opportunities and threats in order to create a direction that emanates from top management. Information about the past and present, and the ability to forecast the future is vital to strategy formation. Successful practices strive to understand their current environment and to create a unique vision with result-oriented goals which will take the practice from where it is now to where it should go. The goal of a successful practice is to define and then achieve the purpose of the practice.

Strategic plans can serve two very different purposes. First and foremost, a strategic plan is used within the practice to guide

An Effective Strategic Plan

in building it into what you want to have. Second, a strategic plan can be used in conjunction with the marketing plan and financial plan to obtain financial backing from investors.

A strategic plan need not be a complex or lengthy document. In most cases, the strategic plan can be two or three typewritten pages in length. The key to creating an effective strategic plan is to thoroughly analyze the current healthcare environment and define the practice that you want to establish (for new practices) or evolve into (for existing practices), write the plan down on paper, and then implement it. This process helps communicate to partners and staff the definition, purpose, vision, and the comprehensive plan that will be deliberately and consistently pursued to accomplish your mission. A strategic plan gives you the ability to see the forest and not just the trees.

In creating a strategic plan, you provide the framework and a strong sense of direction to the practice. That allows you to focus precious resources towards specific goals of the practice and provides you with a formal, step-by-step, long-range approach to accomplishing those goals.

The strategic plan is not a document that is set on a shelf and forgotten. An effective strategic plan is the blueprint to building a practice. You should put a great deal of thought into creating the plan, communicating its contents, and then striving to accomplish its goals. Once created, the strategic plan is the foundation of your practice and should only be changed for compelling reasons such as a competitive threat, environmental changes, or trends in purchasing behavior. Review the strategic plan once a year, as your environment changes, making periodic reappraisal and fine-tuning adjustments if necessary. This helps ensure that the practice avoids complacency and affirms that it is in the right business and achieving the desired results. Imaginative strategy formulation and reformulation when your environment changes is the key to out-performing your competition.

The strategic plan should consist of the following:
- Mission Statement
- Target Markets

An Effective Strategic Plan

- Competitive Analysis
- Strengths, Weaknesses, Opportunities, and Threats
- Goals of the Practice

The following chapters will explain each of these components.

CHAPTER 1
Mission Statement

"To know what a business is we have to start with its purpose. Its purpose must lie outside of the business itself. In fact, it must lie in society since business enterprise is an organ of society. There is only one valid definition of business purpose: to create a customer."
–Peter Drucker

"Success is a product of unremitting attention to purpose."
–Benjamin Disraeli

"Strategic planning is worthless — unless there is first a strategic vision."
–John Naisbitt

The **mission statement** is one sentence that defines the long term vision of what the practice seeks to be and the markets it seeks to service. It should answer the question, "What is the purpose of your practice?" The mission statement describes what you want your practice to be, not what it could be.

While the mission statement is a single sentence, it is critical because it expresses the ultimate goal of your practice. It is the reason that you are in practice. Furthermore, everything the practice accomplishes is done in support of the mission statement.

By defining the mission statement in specific terms, you will be able to focus precious resources more efficiently and

13

An Effective Strategic Plan

effectively. The following questions can help define mission of your practice.
- What type of pain classes are you going to treat (e.g. acute, chronic, cancer)?
- Will your approach be multi-discipline or single specialty? If it is single specialty, will you refer to other specialists?
- Who will be providing the services — anesthesiologists, fellowship trained pain management anesthesiologists, and/or other physicians, such as orthopedics, physical medicine and rehabilitation, neurology, neurosurgery, etc?
- Will the practice require physicians to be board certified or board eligible?
- Will you employ ancillary providers such as physical therapists, occupational therapists, psychologists, etc., or will these services be available only via referral?
- What image do you want in the market? The market is the set of all actual and potential target buyers (medical community, insurance companies, patients, employers, etc.)?

Once these questions have been answered, you should be ready to write a mission statement. Some examples of mission statements are as follows:
- To establish eminence in the field of pain management by providing quality, comprehensive, and cost-effective medical care by fellowship trained, board certified pain management anesthesiologists for the treatment of patients who suffer from acute, chronic, and cancer pain disorders.
- To create a comprehensive, multi-disciplinary pain management program that includes physical therapy, anesthesia pain management, behavior modification, and orthopedic surgery for the treatment of chronic back pain.
- To create a comprehensive cancer treatment center that provides services in chemotherapy, radiation oncology, pain management, home health services, and

psychiatric services, that will become the standard of excellence for the treatment of cancer in the community.
- To provide cost-effective pain management services by anesthesiologists who are trained in pain management for the treatment of acute, chronic, and cancer pain disorders as requested by referring physicians.

As you can see from the above mission statements, the practices that are created to accomplish these missions will be very different. The mission statement is a unique aim that sets one practice apart from other practices by defining the nature and character of what you want to ultimately accomplish in your practice.

An Effective Strategic Plan

CHAPTER 2
Target Markets

*"Success follows doing what you want to do.
There is no other way to be successful."*
–Malcolm Forbes

*"You've got to take the initiative and play your game.
In a decisive set, confidence is the difference."*
–Chris Evert

The mission statement defines the ultimate goal of the practice. The **target market** defines which markets you want to serve with your goal. A target market is a set of customers whose needs and wants the practice plans to satisfy (see pages 33-35 for the definition of needs and wants). A practice should have multiple sets of target markets.

The mission statement answers the question "What is the purpose of your practice?" The target market definition answers the question, "Who are your customers?" or, "Whom do you want as your customers?"

There are several good reasons why a practice should define its target markets. First, your target markets will be used in tailoring your marketing efforts to obtain the practice that you want. These are the people who you want to reach when you are advertising your practice.

Target Markets

Second, the composition of your target markets helps to ensure that there is enough population in your community to support the defined practice.

Third, if you are part of a group of physicians, you can use your target markets to help you define the services that you are going to provide, and also to obtain agreement and commitment in the practice for serving these target markets. For example, let's assume that one physician in a group wants to implant dorsal column stimulators and the rest of the physicians in the same group do not. Then the group must answer several questions. Should a dorsal column stimulator be implanted in a patient if only one member of the group is willing to treat that patient? How will call be handled for the dorsal column stimulator patient? What happens if the physician leaves the group and no other physician in the group wants to or feels qualified to take over the care of the patient? While these situations might not seem necessary to discuss at first, it is better to work out these fundamentals before there is a problem. Once the group has entered into the care of a patient, some managed care companies will require that the group continue to support the patient as long as the device is implanted.

Fourth, knowing your target markets can assist you in recruiting physicians who are interested in pursuing a similar practice. Your definition of target markets tells the recruit: "This is who is served in this practice."

When defining your target markets it is very important that you keep in mind that you define the practice that you want.

There are many ways to group potential customers into target markets. A target market may be defined by demographic characteristics such as gender or age (pediatric, adults, or geriatric) patients. A target market can also be defined by identifying the list of diseases and conditions you want to treat, such as back pain, cancer, headaches, or shingles. A target market can also be a group of doctors in a particular specialty from whom you would like to receive referrals, such as orthopedics, neurosurgery, oncology, or a group of nurses who are employed by workers compensation companies as caseworkers. A target

An Effective Strategic Plan

market also can be a managed care company whose policyholders you would like to have as patients.

You can define as many target markets as you want to serve; however, you need to be sure that you have the skill set and resources to serve the markets that are targeted. The following questions will be helpful in defining target markets:

- What is the age and gender of the patients that you want to treat (e.g. men, women, pediatric, adults, geriatric)?
- What diseases do you want to treat (e.g. cancer, back pain, head and neck pain, complex regional pain syndrome (formerly called reflex sympathetic dystrophy), shingles, neuralgia, headaches, joint pain, arthritis, phantom limb pain, fractured rib pain, compression fracture pain, etc.)?
- What procedures are you going to perform (trigger points, cervical epidural, thoracic epidural, lumbar epidural, caudal epidural, occipital nerve block, intercostal nerve block, injection major joint, ilionguinal nerve block, facet, stellate ganglion nerve block, celiac plexus nerve block, etc.)?
- Will you perform most of your procedures with or without fluoroscopy? Will you always perform neurolytics with fluoroscopy?
- Are you going to implant subarachnoid or epidural catheters with reservoirs and/or pumps, dorsal column stimulators, and/or perform radiofrequency neurolysis?
- What will be the policy toward narcotics? Do you want to treat patients with chronic benign pain with long-term narcotics administration? Will the prescription of narcotics be limited to cancer pain patients?
- In what specialties are your target physician referral sources (e.g. internal medicine, family practice, oncology, orthopedics, physical medicine and rehabilitation, neurosurgery, neurology)?
- Which are the workers compensation insurance companies that could be a source for referrals?
- Which are the managed care companies that could be a source for referrals?

Target Markets

- Who are the caseworkers (such as nurses) who are employed by workers compensation companies to oversee the medical care administered to employees who are injured at work that could be a source for referrals?
- Do you want to target the general public?
- Are there employers in your market who have a large number of employees who might suffer from acute or chronic pain disorders or have work-related injuries?
- Are there hospitals or surgery centers that need or would welcome pain management services and assist in promoting your practice?

Once the target markets are defined, then you need to understand how large each market is and what the trends are within each market. This information indicates whether or not it is economically feasible to create a practice for this target market today and in the future.

For example, you may want to target geriatric patients (defined as patients who are over the age of 65). Let's assume that there are 125,000 people over the age of 65 in your community and that their population is growing at five percent per year. This information indicates that there is a base of patients that is statistically large enough and growing at a rate significant enough to support a geriatric pain management practice in your community now and in the future.

In another example, let's assume that you want to treat pediatric cancer pain exclusively. If this is your goal and you are in a small community, you may find that there are not enough patients in this target market to economically support the practice. Let's assume that the number of pediatric cancer patients in the community is less than 50 patients per year, and it is decreasing at a rate of three percent per year. This indicates that it is not feasible to build a profitable pediatric cancer pain management practice in your community. You many need to relocate to a larger community or expand your practice to other target markets.

Knowing the target market size and growth will allow you to better forecast the need for your services and project growth rates

An Effective Strategic Plan

that are realistic. In order to find out information on the size of a target market, you can often find reference publications from the following information sources:

- The local library.
- The local Chamber of Commerce can supply information on the major employers in the community and the demographics of the population including population size, age, educational level, and income. Often this information can be provided by zip code. This allows you to better quantify the demographics of a specific location within the community.
- The Department of Insurance in your state can supply a list of managed care companies and workers compensation insurance companies that are licensed to do business in your state.
- Large managed care companies may be willing to share demographic and health information on their set of policyholders.
- Local hospitals will sometimes share their market research on the demographics of the community and their patient base.
- Major employers will sometimes share the number of employees and their disability statistics, age, sex, and income.
- Local newspapers and radio and television stations can provide information on the demographics of their customers.
- The Medical Group Management Association (MGMA 104 Inverness Terrace East, Englewood, Colorado 80112) can supply a wide range of books and articles on medical practices.
- The National Center for Health Statistics (U.S. Department of Health and Human Services, 370 East-West Highway, Hattsville, Maryland 20782) can supply information on the population, age, extent and nature of illness, and disability for your community.
- The American Medical Association (AMA, 535 North Dearborn, Chicago, Illinois 60610) can supply a wide variety of information on medical practices.

Target Markets

- The Superintendent of Documents, (U.S. Government Printing Office, Washington, D.C. 20402) can supply a wide variety of information on population, income, disability, health and nutrition, education, and the labor force in your community.

The main reason to understand the demographics of the target market is to help ensure that the target market is statistically significant to support your practice now and in the future. Knowing the demographics of the market can assist in developing realistic and obtainable goals.

You can also analyze the amount of customers that you serve in a given target market as a percent of the total population. This is referred to as market share. For example, let's assume you have identified the population of 65 or older in your community as a target market. You know that there are 125,000 people over the age of 65 in the community. After two years practicing pain management, you have treated 625 of these patients. Then your market share is one half of one percent of the population over 65.

The more information that you have the better your analysis can be. For example, let's assume you know that of the 125,000 people over the age of 65 in your community, only 10 percent, or 12,500 people, will seek treatment for an acute or chronic pain disorder in any given year. In the same two-year period, approximately 25,000 of the people 65 and over in your community will seek pain management services. Then you know that your market share for the 625 patients that were treated during the two-year period was two and one-half percent of the market. You can then use this information to develop strategies to obtain the other 97.5 percent of the business that was served by your direct competitors or by other healthcare providers who do not specialize in pain management.

An Effective Strategic Plan

CHAPTER 3
Competitive Analysis

"Every morning in Africa a gazelle wakes up. It knows it must run faster than the fastest lion or it will be killed. Every morning a lion wakes up also. It knows that is must outrun the slowest gazelle or it will starve to death. It doesn't matter whether you are the lion or the gazelle. When the sun comes up you had better be running."
–Anonymous

To fully understand the market, you need to understand the dynamics of your competition and then create the strategies that will differentiate you from your competition. To understand the competition, it will be helpful to ask the following questions:

- Who are they? What are their qualifications? In what specialty are they trained? Are they board certified? Are they board certified in pain management?
- What services are they providing? Where are they providing services? Do you know or believe that they may be expanding services and/or locations?
- How are their services priced?
- How do they get their business? What doctors refer to them? How loyal are their referring doctors?
- Who are their target markets? What is their market share and current growth rate?
- Do they have contracts with major and/or significant managed care companies in the market? Do they have an exclusive contract with managed care companies?

Competitive Analysis

- Do they have an exclusive contract to provide services at a given location (i.e. a hospital or surgery center)?
- What is the geographical area that they serve? It is growing or shrinking?
- How are they perceived in the market? Are they considered a leader or a follower? How effective is their marketing and advertising?
- How well does their business office operate?
- How well does their clinical office operate?
- What are their strengths? What are their weaknesses?
- Are they vulnerable?
- How successful are they in executing their strategy?
- How have they responded to changes in economic conditions and market trends?
- What will they most likely do in the future? How will they react to your practice's introduction or enhancement of available pain management services?

An understanding of the competitor's business strategy is fundamental to developing a winning strategy. By understanding the competition you can answer the question, "How can my practice better serve the market?" Later, when you define your services and develop your marketing plan, you will formulate the strategies that will help you answer this question.

Many physicians neglect to ask these questions, perhaps because they feel that their service is superior or that there will be plenty of patients for all competitors. However, it is difficult to outmaneuver the competition without first understanding what they are doing in the marketplace. Ignoring or underestimating the competition can be a fatal mistake to your practice.

CHAPTER 4
SWOT

"We are all continually faced with a series of great opportunities brilliantly disguised as insoluble problems."
–John W. Gardner

"To improve the golden moment of opportunity, and catch the good that is within our reach, is the great art of life."
–William James

Many business books refer to the process of analyzing the practice as doing a **"SWOT" analysis.** SWOT is an acronym for a business' strengths, weakness, opportunities, and threats. When identifying strengths and weakness, think of every aspect of the internal operations of the practice from the clinical procedures to the business office operations. A concise and honest appraisal of your practice's strengths and weaknesses will greatly assist in seeking and developing opportunities which will allow you to capitalize on your strengths and improve your weaknesses.

To begin, focus internally on what makes you the best in serving your target markets. Then identify the areas where you most need to improve. Next, look at the industry and other external market factors that may present opportunities or threats to your practice. When you identify a strength of your practice and find that your competition either does not have this strength or performs it poorly, then you have found an opportunity. When you find an item that could negatively impact your practice, then you have found a threat. The following questions will be helpful in identifying your strength, weaknesses, opportunities, and threats.

Strengths

- Are you better trained than your competitors? Are you Board Certified? Are you fellowship trained in pain management?
- What are the strengths in your clinical operations?
- Do you have or can you get managed care contracts with the key managed care companies in your market?
- Are there innovative services that you can offer that your competition does not have?
- Can you provide service more rapidly than your competition without sacrificing patient care?
- Can you achieve cost-efficiencies that will maximize profit without negatively impacting patient care?
- Can you provide better service and better patient care than your competitors?
- Is your office building visible, easily accessible, and centrally located?
- Do you have multiple locations to accommodate patient's needs?
- Do you market your services to your target markets more effectively than your competition?
- Do you know how to effectively bill and get paid for your services?
- What strengths are in your internal business operations?
- Do you have a tracking system so that you know who refers patients? Are you using this information to protect and increase your business?
- Do you have patient loyalty?
- Do you have referring physician loyalty?
- Do you have effective internal management?
- Do you have above average profitability?

An Effective Strategic Plan

- Do you have adequate financial resources?

Weaknesses

- Do you have a clear strategic direction? Do you and your employees understand your mission and target markets?
- Do you have a weak market image? Do you have the marketing skills to create an image and obtain referrals?
- Do you have the financial resources to build a successful pain practice? Are you willing to commit the financial resources to building this pain management practice?
- Are you spreading your physicians too thin by asking them to cover both the operating room and pain management?
- Does your group agree that starting a pain practice is a good idea?
- What are the weaknesses in your clinical operations?
- What are the weaknesses in your internal business operations?
- Are you plagued with internal operating problems?

Opportunities

- Can you create a market for pain management services?
- Do you offer services that your competitors do not offer?
- Who controls the referral of patients and can you change the referral patterns?
- Are your competitors complacent or are they growing their market share?
- Are there any competitors who are planning to exit from the market?
- Are the demographics of your community changing so that there will be an increase in demand for pain management services?

Threats

- Are you a participating provider with the key managed care companies? Do your competitors have exclusive contracts that will prevent you from becoming a participating provider?
- Will you be able to negotiate with managed care companies for reimbursement levels that will allow your practice to be profitable?
- Can your practice be profitable serving Medicare and Medicaid patients?
- Can you get on staff at the hospitals and/or surgery centers of your choice? Do your competitors have exclusive staff privileges at hospitals and surgery centers that will limit your ability to obtain staff privileges?
- Will there be regulatory influences and government policy changes that will effect pain management?
- Where is pain management headed? Are there fundamental changes in the industry that will affect your practice?
- Are there any competitors who are planning to enter the market?
- Are there any substitute products or services that can replace your services?
- Do you use correctly code claims to limit the risk of Medicare, Medicaid, and/or other insurance audit or fraud?
- Do you utilize generally accepted accounting practices to limit the risk of an IRS audit or fraud?
- Does your practice have any relationships with referring doctors that violate the Federal Anti-Kickback Statute of the Ethics in Patient Referrals Act (STARK). See pages 115-119.

The SWOT analysis helps you understand where you are now in the business world. You will use this information to help develop a successful marketing plan, one that will help you attain your goals.

CHAPTER 5
Goals of the Practice

"If you really know what things you want out of life, it's amazing how opportunities will come to enable you to carry them out."
–John M. Goddard

"Procrastination is a close relative of incompetence and a handmaiden of inefficiency."
–Alec MacKenzie

Defining your goals answers the question, "What do I want to accomplish in my practice?" A goal should be realistic and stated in specific, concrete terms against which actual results can be easily measured. *Specific goals transform strategy into results-oriented measurable commitments.*

Goals consist of three elements:
- Subject — What is the subject area of your goal?
- Time frame — When do you want to accomplish the goal?
- Measurement — How much to you want to accomplish?

In order to define a goal begin by focusing on the mission statement, which will help you define the **subject** of the goals that you want to accomplish. Then review the SWOT analysis for the factors that may effect your ability to succeed. Do you

Goals of the Practice

have internal strengths or weakness that could become a goal? Are there opportunities or threats that could become a goal?

It is important that the goals that you define have a **time frame.** The time frame gives you a sense of urgency to accomplish a goal. Without a time frame, goals can easily be left unaccomplished. For example the goal of "Someday the practice will have 1000 new patients per year," is common, but all too often someday never arrives.

Goals must also have realistic **measurements;** both internal and external factors will effect how much you can realistically achieve. Internal factors have to do with your practice's ability to accomplish goals. External factors have to do with what your competitors, managed care companies, and/or the government are doing which may effect your ability or speed to accomplish your goals.

Review goals with staff members to obtain their input and assessment. When staff members are involved in shared decision making and goal-setting, they are more likely to commit to accomplish the goals. Staff members who are given authority and responsibility to accomplish goals have higher job satisfaction because they feel valued and trusted. Further, staff members also gain a sense of control, ownership, pride, and involvement in the success of the practice. Some examples of goals are:

- To obtain an average of 10 new patients per week during the first year in practice.
- To receive new patient referrals from at least 100 different physicians by the end of the first year.
- To have at least 20 physicians by the end of the year who refer at least one patient per month.
- To increase the number of new patients per year at a rate of 20 percent annually.
- To hire a second pain management physician by the end of the second year of practice.
- To maintain an overhead expense ratio which does not exceed 40 percent of the gross charges of the practice.
- To establish a reputation for on-time service. New patients will not wait more than three business days to

An Effective Strategic Plan

obtain a first time appointment. Patients will not wait more than 15 minutes in the reception area before being seen by a physician.
- To establish a reputation for outstanding patient care measured by obtaining an average total score of 25 or less on a patient satisfaction survey (see pages 38-43 for information on the patient satisfaction survey).
- To publish two articles on pain management annually.

Once your goals are defined, you need to ask the following questions:
- Are the goals realistic and obtainable?
- Are there any factors that would aid or hinder you in your pursuit of these goals?
- Can you realistically expect to achieve your goals, considering the talent, resources, and limitations of your practice?

Once you have defined realistic goals of the practice, the entire practice should focus on pursuing and obtaining these goals. Performance appraisals, promotions, and bonuses should be based upon accomplishing the goals. Those unwilling or unable to commit themselves to the goals after counseling and coaching should be asked to leave the practice. Practices that focus on rewarding positive results, not on punishing mistakes, and that reward staff and physicians verbally and economically will foster a culture that nurtures success.

THE KEYS TO SUCCESSFUL MARKETING

BOOK II
The Keys to Successful Marketing

*"Business has only two basic functions –
marketing and innovation."*
–Peter Drucker

*"There are three types of companies. Those who
make things happen. Those who watch things happen.
Those who wonder what happened."*
–Anonymous

    The term "marketing" has many different meanings to many different people. Marketing is the process of satisfying needs and wants of target markets through the creation of public awareness of products and services that are offered by the practice. Marketing involves needs assessment, marketing research, service development, pricing, timing, packaging, advertising, selling, public relations, and test marketing. Each of these marketing elements will be described in this section.

    The ultimate goal of marketing is to convert strategy into results. It is the means to the end. The Marketing Plan answers the question, "How are you going to achieve the mission and goals of your practice?" Knowledge of the marketing elements discussed in this section are necessary to write and implement an effective marketing plan (see pages 141-148 for an example of a marketing plan).

CHAPTER 1
Needs Assessment

"A business is not defined by the company's name, statutes, or articles of corporation. It is defined by the want the customer satisfies when he buys a product or service. To satisfy the customer is the mission and purpose of every business. . . . What the customer sees, thinks, believes, and wants, at any given time, must be accepted by management as an objective fact . . ."
–Peter Drucker

"Truth has to fall on fertile soil."
–Paula D'Arcy

The first step in marketing is to understand **the needs and wants of your target markets.** In the strategic plan, potential customers are defined as your target markets. The target markets could be, but are not limited to, patients, referring physicians, managed care companies, and other third-party payers such as workers compensation insurance companies. When you create the marketing plan, you ask, "What do the target markets need and want?"

A need is defined as a fundamental item which when left unsatisfied creates a state of deprivation. Human beings have many needs. They include air, water, food, clothing, warmth, safety and compassion. When a need is not satisfied the person will be unhappy. Unhappy people will do one of do one of two things — try to satisfy the need or try to eliminate the need.

33

The Keys to Successful Marketing

A want is defined as an expression of a human need. For example a person is thirsty. The thirst is a need that can be satisfied by drinking any one of a variety of liquids. The marketer's job is to create the want for a product to satisfy the need. If you are selling bottled water, your goal is to create a want for your brand of bottled water. If you are selling soda, your goal is to create a want for your brand of soda. Another example is a person who has back pain. The back pain is a need that can be satisfied by treatment through an orthopedic surgeon or a pain management physician. The marketer's job is to create the want for the patient, perhaps via the referring doctor, to seek treatment by not only a pain management physician, but more specially, at your pain management practice.

Different target markets have different needs, and a given target market may have many needs. *Successful practices understand what their target markets want and need. They detect changes and trends in purchasing behavior and respond to them quickly.* Some examples of needs are as follows:

- A pain patient's need is to resolve the underlying pain disorder and to be pain-free.
- A pain patient's need is for human compassion and understanding about the pain complaint.
- A pain patient's need is for prompt and professional service.
- A referring physician's need is to manage risk by referring patients to another physician who is trained to resolve patients' pain complaints.
- A referring physician's need is to know what the underlying pain disorder is and how the pain disorder will be treated.
- A referring physician's need is to maintain overall control of the patient's care.
- A managed care company's need is to provide cost-effective health coverage to insured policyholders.
- A workers' compensation insurance company's need is to get the insured patient back to work as soon as possible.

Needs Assessment

Sometimes, you will not know your target market's needs and wants. *In order to find out, conduct market research.*

CHAPTER 2
Market Research

"The best way for a firm to be lucky is to make its own luck. That requires knowing what makes a business successful."
–Theodore Levitt

"To manage a business well is to manage its future; and to manage its future is to manage information."
–Marion Harper, Jr.

Market research is the process of determining the needs and wants of a target market. In many cases it is the straightforward accumulation of data available from assessing your practice or in published sources. In some cases, you will want to conduct a **market survey** of your target markets. For example you could:
- Survey current and former patients to find out what experiences that they had with your practice so you can improve your services.
- Survey potential patients to find out what they need and want from a pain management physician.
- Survey both doctors who have and have not referred patients to you who are in your target market to find out what they want from a pain management service.
- Survey nurses who are employed by workers' compensation insurance companies to find out what they want from a pain management service.

Market Research

- Survey the major insurance and managed care companies in your community to find out what they want from a pain management service.

If you are in an existing practice, you may be able to gain insight into your markets' needs and wants by assessing your practice. You may already know the following information:

- Who are the physicians who refer patients?
- In what specialties are the physicians who refer patients?
- What is the market share by referring physician specialty? The market share is a percentage of the total market that you currently serve. For example, let's assume that there are 100 orthopedic surgeons in your community and that 20 have referred patients, then you know that 20 percent of the orthopedic surgeons have referred patients.
- What is the market share by each referring doctor? For example, let's assume that an orthopedic surgeon refers a total of 100 patients to pain specialists each year and that 40 patients were referred to you. Then your market share of the doctor's total referrals is 40 percent.
- What pain disorders do you currently treat?
- What is your market share by pain disorder? For example, if you know that 10,000 patients were treated for back pain in your community, and you treated 100 patients, then your market share is one percent of the total back pain patients.
- What are the results of your patient satisfaction surveys (see pages 38-43 for information on patient satisfaction surveys)? Were the patients needs and wants satisfied, or do you have areas where you need to improve?
- What are the results of your referring doctors' surveys (see pages 44-46 for information on referring doctor surveys)? Were the referring physicians' needs and wants satisfied, or do you have areas where you need to improve?
- What were the results of other surveys that you may have conducted on other target markets? Were the

The Keys to Successful Marketing

target markets needs and wants satisfied, or do you have areas where you need to improve?

Once you have identified the needs and wants of the target markets, you can develop **products and services** to satisfy their needs and wants.

Satisfaction Surveys

> "Rule 1. The customer is always right.
> Rule 2. If the customer is wrong, reread Rule 1."
> –Stew Leonard

> "There is only one boss. The customer. And he can fire everybody in the company, from the chairman on down, simply by spending his money somewhere else."
> –Sam Walton

> "An organization, however efficient and well-administered it may be, simply cannot be successful or outstanding or a winner if it is doing the wrong things."
> –Thompson and Strickland

A satisfaction survey is unique to each practice because it will measure what you want to know from a member of your target market about your practice. The purpose of a survey is to measure results and identify complaints that your target markets have with your practice. Once you have obtained responses, you should carefully study them and make all of the reasonable improvements that are suggested.

It is critical to your long-term success that you satisfy the needs and wants of your target markets. This does not mean giving the patient, managed care company, or referring physician everything that they ask for. It does mean providing the proper expectation, communication, and education about the patient's health, and the understanding of their healthcare plan, recommended protocols, and the provision of appropriate care in a timely, efficient, and professional manner.

It is much easier and cost-effective to keep an existing client in your target market than it is to recruit and obtain a new individual. There is an old saying: "It costs less to do it right the first time than it does to do it over."

The long-term goal of your practice is to maintain the business that you have and increase new business. The way to increase your practice's business is to solve any obstacles that may exist between a member of your target group, (e.g. patient, referring doctor, managed care company, etc.) and your ability to provide a service which satisfies their needs. The survey is one mechanism that allows you to monitor how well you are doing at keeping the business that you have and at eliminating problems.

Unhappy clients are more likely to communicate their dissatisfaction than happy clients are to communicate their satisfaction, but often they do not tell you of their unhappiness unless you ask. If you have not asked, then to whom are these unhappy people communicating their dissatisfaction? In many cases unhappy clients tell their friends, family members, doctors, and hospital personnel that they did not like the services that you provided. This negative feedback can ruin your reputation in the community.

If you hear a complaint, you need to take corrective action. In many cases the corrective action not only benefits the person who was unsatisfied, but other people who will in the future use your services. Often a person's loyalty is increased if they know that their complaint was heard and the corrective action was taken. But if you don't hear the complaint, or worse, if you hear the complaint and do nothing about it, the person's dissatisfaction is increased. A dissatisfied person will tell an average of nine other people of their experience. But a successfully handled complaint will not only restore these nine potentially lost opportunities, but more than likely it will also change the person who complained into an advocate for your services.

A complaint is a business opportunity to improve your services. Instead of discouraging complaints, the office personnel along with the patient satisfaction survey should make it easy to register complaints.

The Keys to Successful Marketing

To develop a positive long-term relationship with members of your target markets you need to provide high quality service and the ability to satisfy their needs completely. *Satisfied people will tell other people of their experiences and your practice will grow.*

The survey should be professional, clear, and concisely worded so that the person being surveyed can respond quickly. As a general rule, limit the survey to 20 or less questions. It is also often very helpful to allow the person being surveyed space to comment in a free-form text. Ask the person being surveyed to identify themselves by stating, "If you have a specific complaint and you would like for us to call you, please give us your name and phone number at the bottom of the survey, and we'll get back to you as soon as possible." If you use this statement, be sure that the practice commits sufficient resources to telephone the people who identified themselves within a few days of receiving their complaint.

The following pages show two examples of target market surveys: the first is a patient satisfaction survey and the second is a referring doctor satisfaction survey.

Market Research

Example of a Patient Satisfaction Survey

NEW TOWN PAIN INSTITUTE
Your Opinion Counts

We invite you to help us improve our services to you. Please take a few minutes to complete this brief survey. If you have a specific complaint and you would like for us to call you, please write your name and phone number on the bottom of the survey, and we'll get back to you as soon as possible. We appreciate your opinion and thank you for your patronage.

Appointment Date: _____

Physician seen (check one):

❏ David M. Jones, M.D.   ❏ Mary C. Smith, M.D.

Please indicate your response to the following questions by circling the appropriate number according to this scale:

  1 = Strongly Agree 2 = Agree 3 = Don't Know
  4 = Disagree 5 = Strongly Disagree

---

a. It was easy to reach The New Town Pain Institute by phone.

  1   2   3   4   5

b. I was able to get an appointment at The New Town Pain Institute within a reasonable amount of time.

  1   2   3   4   5

c. I was seen promptly by the physician after I arrived at The New Town Pain Institute.

  1   2   3   4   5

d. The New Town Pain Institute office location was convenient to reach.

  1   2   3   4   5

e. The New Town Pain Institute office was clean and pleasant.

  1   2   3   4   5

The Keys to Successful Marketing

    f. The New Town Pain Institute parking was convenient.
        1   2   3   4   5

    g. The employees at The New Town Pain Institute were professional and courteous both in person and on the telephone.
        1   2   3   4   5

    h. The physician at The New Town Pain Institute was professional and courteous.
        1   2   3   4   5

    i. The New Town Pain Institute physician spent an adequate amount of time talking to me and examining me during the appointment.
        1   2   3   4   5

    j. The New Town Pain Institute physician adequately explained my diagnosis, treatment options, and prescriptions, if any.
        1   2   3   4   5

    k. I feel that the physician and employees of The New Town Pain Institute understand my pain complaint and are compassionate.
        1   2   3   4   5

    l. I selected The New Town Pain Institute because they were listed on my health insurance plan as a provider.
        1   2   3   4   5

    m. The charges on my bill were reasonable for the services that I received from The New Town Pain Institute.
        1   2   3   4   5

    n I feel satisfied with the health care that I received at The New Town Pain Institute.
        1   2   3   4   5

    o. I would recommend The New Town Pain Institute to a friend or family member.
        1   2   3   4   5

Market Research

Please comment:
_____
_____
_____
_____
_____
_____
_____

Name (optional):
_____

Would you like for us to call you?   ❑ Yes ❑ No
If yes, phone number where you can be reached:
days _____
evenings _____

The Keys to Successful Marketing

Example of a Reffering Physician Survey

NEW TOWN PAIN INSTITUTE
Your Opinion Counts

We invite you to help us improve our service to you. Please take a few minutes to complete this brief survey. If you have a specific complaint and you would like for us to call you, please write your name and phone number on the bottom of the survey, and we'll get back to you as soon as possible. We appreciate your opinion and thank you for your referrals.

Please indicate your response to the following questions by circling the appropriate number according to this scale:

1 = Strongly Agree 2 = Agree 3 = Don't Know
4 = Disagree 5 = Strongly Disagree

a. I prefer to have my patients seen by Dr. David M. Jones.
    1   2   3   4   5

b. I prefer to have my patients seen by Dr. Mary C. Smith.
    1   2   3   4   5

c. I feel that both physicians at The New Town Pain Institute provide the same level and quality of care.
    1   2   3   4   5

d. I refer my patients to The New Town Pain Institute because they participate with the managed care plans that my patients are enrolled in.
    1   2   3   4   5

e. I refer my patients to The New Town Pain Institute because my patients request to be referred there.
    1   2   3   4   5

Market Research

f. I refer my patients to The New Town Pain Institute because they offer the best pain management program in New Town.

    1   2   3   4   5

g. It was easy to refer a patient to The New Town Pain Institute.

    1   2   3   4   5

h. The employees at The New Town Pain Institute were professional and courteous to my employees and to me on both the telephone and in person.

    1   2   3   4   5

I. I did not have to wait long to get an appointment for my patient with The New Town Pain Institute.

    1   2   3   4   5

J. The New Town Pain Institute physician sent me a letter that clearly explained the patient's diagnosis, treatment options, and prescriptions, if any.

    1   2   3   4   5

k. The New Town Pain Institute's correspondence was timely.

    1   2   3   4   5

l. I was kept informed of my patient's on-going treatment and progress.

    1   2   3   4   5

m. My patients were appropriately returned back to me for follow-up care.

    1   2   3   4   5

n. My telephone calls to The New Town Pain Institute physicians were promptly returned.

    1   2   3   4   5

0. I believe that my patients feel that billed charges were reasonable for the services they received from The New Town Pain Institute.

The Keys to Successful Marketing

        1   2   3   4   5

p. Overall, I feel satisfied with the health care that was provided to my patients by The New Town Pain Institute.

        1   2   3   4   5

q. I will continue to refer patients to The New Town Pain Institute.

        1   2   3   4   5

Please comment:

_____
_____
_____
_____
_____
_____
_____

Name (optional):

_____

Would you like for us to call you?   ❑ Yes ❑ No

If yes, phone number where you can be reached:

days _____

evenings _____

CHAPTER 3
Creating the "Want" for Your Practice

"Markets are not created by God, nature, or economic forces but by businessmen."
–Peter Drucker

Many physicians are capable of resolving underlying pain disorders and getting the patient to a pain-free state. *Your goal in marketing your practice is to create the "want" for the patients to come to your practice, and for physicians and managed care companies to refer patients to your practice.*

Physicians may have many choices when referring a pain patient; for example, a back pain patient could be referred to an orthopedic surgeon, neurosurgeon, physical medicine and rehabilitation physician, or a pain management physician. If the patient is referred to a pain management physician, there may also be many choices of groups to which the physician can refer. In addition, managed care companies have many participating providers to whom they will refer patients. Your goal in marketing your practice is to create the want for physicians and the managed care companies to refer or help direct the patient to your practice. You can create the want for your practice by:

- Developing services that meet the needs and wants of your target markets.
- Being the best. Create a history of successfully resolving patients' pain complaints.

The Keys to Successful Marketing

- Treating your target markets ethically and with respect, integrity, and honesty.
- Establishing reasonable prices for your services and adhering to ethical billing practices.
- Creating awareness for your practice through advertising and selling.
- Building external creditability through promotional activities and public relations.

The following chapters will discuss how you can create a want for your practice.

CHAPTER 4
Service Development

"People no longer buy shoes to keep their feet warm and dry. They buy them because of the way the shoes make them feel — masculine, feminine, rugged, different, sophisticated, young, glamorous, "in. . ." Buying shoes has become an emotional experience. Our business is selling excitement rather than shoes."
–Francis C. Rooney

"You have to learn the rules of the game. And then play better than everyone else."
–Diane Feinstein

"Give the lady what she wants."
–W. C. Fields

To be successful in pain management, you must change your mind-set from an operating room mentality to a service-oriented referral-based mentality. In the operating room, patients are sent to you because a surgeon has scheduled a procedure. *To be successful in pain management, you must develop an on-going stream of patients by providing services that satisfy the needs and/or wants of your target markets.*

When you see a patient for a consult, office visit, or to perform a procedure, you are providing a service directly to the patient. You are also providing a service when you call or send a

49

The Keys to Successful Marketing

letter to a referring physician or when you treat policyholders of a managed care company.

In order to develop your services, first review the needs and wants of your target groups and then provide the services that satisfy these needs and wants. Some examples of services are as follows:

- The ability to effectively resolve the patient's pain complaint.
- Providing the most advanced medical treatment available for the patient's pain complaint by making a commitment to stay abreast of changes in medical treatment by constantly reading medical literature.
- Participating with Medicare, Medicaid, Workers Compensation, and most managed care and/or insurance company's plans.
- Offering evening and weekend hours.
- Expanding urgent care capability to help limit emergency room use.
- Offering a customer service department.
- Providing patient education on pain disorders and preventative care.
- Providing referral services that are patient-friendly.
- Offering timely appointment availability.
- Offering current magazines in the reception area.
- Promptly seeing and treating patients.
- Treating patients with compassion, professionalism, and a positive attitude.
- Greeting patients in the reception area with a smile.
- Maintaining a clean, state-of-the-art, professional facility.
- Having an office that is centrally located.
- Having more than one location if patient population is geographically disbursed.
- Having reasonable fees for services rendered.
- Always washing hands in front of the patient to convey the perception of cleanliness.

Service Development

- Telephoning physicians who have referred a patient for the first time. Tell them that on routine cases you normally send a letter; however if they prefer, you could telephone them whenever their patient is seen. This process helps to establish a relationship with new referring physicians.
- Telephoning the referring physician when it is prudent due to medical necessity.
- Sending a timely, concise, and accurate letter to the referring physician after seeing the patient for the first time.
- Sending follow-up letters to the referring physician to keep him/her aware of the patient's progress.
- When appropriate and/or at the completion of their pain management treatment, send patients back to the care of the referring physician.
- Maintaining accurate, complete, organized, and neat medical records.
- Maintaining accurate, complete, organized, and neat billing records that are separate from the medical records.
- Sending a timely and accurate claim to managed care companies.
- Sending a timely and accurate statement to the patient.
- Being understanding and willing to work with patients who do not have the ability to pay in full.
- Responding promptly to inquiries from managed care companies regarding the patient's diagnosis and medical treatment.
- Providing managed care companies and referring physicians with summarized anonymous results of the patient satisfaction survey.
- Providing managed care companies and referring physicians with results of the quality assurance outcome data.
- Providing cost-effective case management for managed care companies and workers compensation insurance companies.

The Keys to Successful Marketing

- Taking extra time to discuss patients' care with the workers compensation caseworker.
- Sending copies of medical records to attorneys who request them in a timely manner.
- Giving an accurate and timely deposition for attorneys who request them.
- Giving presentations to local groups on pain management or a specific pain topic.
- Volunteering to answer questions on a radio of TV talk show on pain management or a specific pain topic.

The services that are offered by the practice should meet the individual needs and wants of the target markets of the practice. If a target group has a need or want that is not being satisfied by the practice, remember that the target group can always seek another practice to satisfy that need or want. Moreover, the better that your practice is at providing services to meet the target markets' needs and wants, the more that the practice will be able to differentiate itself from other practices.

Chapter 5
Pricing — Creating a Fee Schedule

"The value of a service, if not fixed in advance, is left to the discretion of the recipient."
–Aristotle

"When it comes time to hang the capitalists, they will compete with each other to sell us the rope at a lower price."
–Lenin

"There is no brand loyalty that two cents off can't overcome."
–Anonymous

The goal of pricing your services is to establish fair market prices for the services rendered. The list of prices that you charge is referred to as a fee schedule. There are several steps to determine a fee schedule, including:
- Identify every procedure that you will perform.
- Obtain the Medicare Fee Schedule.
- Obtain the ASA Relative Value Guide.
- Obtain fee and reimbursement information for your zip code area.
- Analyze the data and draft a fee schedule.
- Perform a reasonableness check and finalize the fee schedule.

The Keys to Successful Marketing

Identify Every Procedure

Procedures are documented by a shorthand common language CPT-4 codes, which stands for *Current Procedural Terminology, Fourth Edition*. These five-digit codes are defined by the American Medical Association and published annually. The most current publication, *The 1998 Physicians Current Procedural Terminology, Fourth Edition,* contains the most detailed CPT-4 descriptions published by any source. Read the CPT-4 book and identify all the procedures that you will be performing. Review annual changes and incorporate them into your procedure list.

Medicare Part B Fee Schedule

Medicare has two parts: Part A is for facilities (hospitals and surgery centers), and Part B is for physician services. Obtain a copy of the current Medicare Part B Fee Schedule published by the U.S. Department of Health and Human Services Health Care Financing Administration (HCFA). It is published annually by the Medicare carrier for your state. For example, the Medicare carrier for the state of Kentucky is AdminiStar Federal, a Subsidiary of Anthem Insurance Companies, Inc. The 1998 Medicare Part B Fee Schedule for the state of Kentucky is entitled *Kentucky Medicare Part B 1998 Participation Program for Physicians with Participation Agreement 1998 Physician Fee Schedule.*

This book contains some introductory information and tables that contain the reimbursement that Medicare will pay, listed by CPT-4 code. Physicians have the option to either participate or not to participate with Medicare. You will need to decide whether or not you want to participate. In 1998, over 80 percent of all physicians participated in the Medicare program. In either case, there are federal laws that govern how much a physician is allowed to charge Medicare participants. If you elect not to participate with Medicare, Medicare will still make payments to you for covered, medically necessary services as long as you

Pricing — Creating a Fee Schedule

have acquired a unique provider number (UPIN). There are several advantages to participating with Medicare:

- Medicare will pay you five percent more than non-participating providers. However, it is important to note that the total amount collected for a non-participating physician (referred to as "the limiting charge") will be five percent greater than the total reimbursement for a participating provider. For example, a lumbar epidural separate procedure, CPT-4 code 62289 in the *1998 Kentucky Medicare Part B Fee Schedule* is as follows:

Procedure Code/Mod	Note	Par Fee Sched	Non-Par Sched	Limiting Charge
62289		96.41	91.59	105.33

A participating physician performing the above procedure would collect 80 percent of $96.41 ($77.13) from Medicare and the remaining 20 percent of $96.41 ($19.28) from the patient. A non-participating physician performing the above procedure would collect 80 percent of $91.59 ($73.28) from Medicare and the difference between the limiting charge of $105.33 and what Medicare paid $32.05 from the patient.

- You will be listed in the Medicare Directory.
- You can submit claims to Medicare electronically via a toll-free number, thus expediting payment to your practice.
- The claims filed on Medicare participants with Medigap coverage (Medicare secondary insurance) will be filed automatically, thus reducing paperwork and labor.

The first eight pages of the *1998 Kentucky Medicare Part B Fee Schedule* contain the "Fact Sheet." The Fact Sheet lists major new and changed Medicare rules and guidelines. While this is helpful information, the Fact Sheet does not contain every Medicare rule, nor does it always contain all of the changes for the current year.

The Keys to Successful Marketing

HCFA defines the fees that Medicare will pay both participating providers and non-participating providers for all covered services. Medicare fees are based upon the RBRVS (resource based relative value system), a system that defines a relative value number for each CPT-4 procedure code based upon the complexity of the procedure relative to other procedures. This number is then multiplied by a dollar conversion factor to determine the Medicare reimbursement amount payable to the provider. This amount, commonly referred to as "the allowable," is shown on the Medicare fee schedule in a column entitled the "Par Fee Sched" (participating provider fee schedule).

HCFA also defines the limiting charge that can be billed a Medicare participant by a non-participating provider. This amount is the maximum that you can receive from a patient if you do not participate with Medicare.

To look up the Medicare allowable for a specific procedure, find the CPT-4 code that corresponds with that procedure. For example, a trigger point injection is CPT-4 code 20550. When you turn to page four of the *1998 Kentucky Medicare Part B Fee Schedule*, you find two lines for CPT-4 code 20550, they are:

Procedure Code/Mod	Note	Par Fee Sched	Non-Par Sched	Limiting Charge
20550		41.43	39.36	45.26
20550	*	35.36	33.59	38.63

There are two lines because a trigger point injection can be performed in either an office or in a facility (hospital or ambulatory surgery center). If the procedure is performed in a facility, the facility will also bill Medicare for the use of the facility. In order to encourage physicians to perform trigger point injections in their offices, there is a five percent reduction in the allowable if the procedure is performed in a place of service other than an office. This reduction is commonly referred to as the site of service reduction. The asterisk which appears in the note column refers to the footnote: "This amount and limiting charge apply

Pricing — Creating a Fee Schedule

when the place of service is a hospital inpatient or outpatient and ambulatory surgical center." When comparing fees, use the first fee listed and not the discounted fee.

Another example is a lumbar epidural separate procedure, CPT-4 code 62289. When you turn to page 33 of the *1998 Kentucky Medicare Part B Fee Schedule*, you find one line for CPT-4 code 62289:

Procedure Code/Mod	Note	Par Fee Sched	Non-Par Sched	Limiting Charge
62289		96.41	91.59	105.33

Since a lumbar epidural separate procedure is rarely performed anywhere except at a facility (hospital or ambulatory surgery center) there is no site of service reduction.

ASA Relative Value

Annually, the American Society of Anesthesiologists (ASA) publishes a relative value guide, the most current being *1998 Relative Value Guide: A Guide for Anesthesia Values*. The *Relative Value Guide* lists the CPT-4 code, a brief description, and a basic unit value for each procedure. The book includes the CPT-4 codes that are used in anesthesia, including pain management. The basic unit value is a number that defines the complexity of a procedure relative to other procedures. For example, a trigger point injection, CPT-4 code 20550, has a relative value of 3, and a lumbar epidural separate procedure, CPT-4 code 62289, has a relative value of 8. Therefore, according to the ASA, a lumbar epidural is over two and one-half times more complex to perform than a trigger point.

The *Relative Value Guide* also contains the diagnosis codes, or ICD-9 codes, that are used in anesthesia, including those codes used for pain management.

The Keys to Successful Marketing

To obtain the *ASA Relative Value Guide*, call the ASA at (847) 825-5586. There is a nominal charge for this book; in 1998, the charge for the book was $15.00. The guide contains only a brief description of the CPT-4 code. For a more complete description refer to the AMA's *The 1998 Physicians Current Procedural Terminology, Fourth Edition.*

Reimbursement Information

There are companies who publish fee and reimbursement information by procedure code (CPT-4 code) for a given zip code area. Fees are the amount that physicians charge for services rendered. Reimbursement is the amount that insurance companies are willing to pay for those services. The best way to find out how much other physicians are charging for their services and how much managed care companies are paying in your zip code area is to purchase an analysis book. One of these companies is Medicode (800-999-4600). For a fee, Medicode will create a *Physician Fee Analyzer Plus* book which is customized for your area and specialty using its database of over 400 million charges. This book contains a list of the CPT-4 codes, a brief description of the CPT-4 code, the average allowable reimbursement paid by an indemnity insurance company, and the 50th, 75th, and 95th percentile of what most physicians charge.

Analyze the Data

Analyze the data while keeping in mind your service goal: to establish fair market prices for the services that you are rendering. Create a spreadsheet that has the following columns:
- CPT-4 code
- Brief description of the CPT-4 code
- Medicare allowable
- ASA relative value unit
- Average indemnity insurance reimbursement amount/low range

Pricing — Creating a Fee Schedule

- Average indemnity insurance reimbursement amount/high range
- 50th percentile of what most physicians charge
- 75h percentile of what most physicians charge
- 95th percentile of what most physicians charge
- 50th percentile of what most physicians charge divided by the ASA relative value unit
- 75h percentile of what most physicians charge divided by the ASA relative value unit
- Proposed fee
- Proposed fee divided by ASA relative value unit
- Proposed fee divided by the 50th percentile of what most physicians charge
- Proposed fee divided by the 75th percentile of what most physicians charge

Then, for each CPT-4 code that you will be performing, input into the column the information described in the column title. The proposed fee can be created using one or all of the following methods:

- **ASA Relative Value Method.** Create a per unit charge that is multiplied by the by the ASA Relative Value Unit amount. For example, let's assume you decide to charge $50 per unit. According to the ASA Relative Value Guide, a trigger point injection, CPT-4 code 20550, has a relative value of 3, and a lumbar epidural separate procedure, CPT-4 code 62289, has a relative value of 8. Using this method, you would charge $150 for a trigger point injection and $400 for a lumbar epidural *(see Figure 1)*.

    Notice that if the proposed fee divided by the 50 percent average of what physician charge is equal to one, then the charge is equal to what most physicians charge. If this number is less than one, then the proposed rate is less than what most physicians' charge. Greater than one means that the proposed fee is more than what most physicians charge. In this example, CPT-4 codes that have a low ASA relative value, such as trigger point in-

FIGURE 1: ASA RELATIVE VALUE METHOD (partial list)

CPT-4 Code	CPT-4 Code Description	Medicare Allowable	ASA Relative Value	Average Indemnity Low	Average Indemnity High	50% Avg. Physician Charge
20550	Injection, tendon sheath, ligament, trigger points, or ganglion cyst	41.43	3	80.30	88.00	78.10
20600	Arthrocentesis, aspiration and/or injection; small joint, bursa or ganlion cyst (e.g. fingers, toes)	38.07	3	73.70	80.30	71.50
20605	Arthrocentesis, aspiration and/or injection; intermediate joint, bursa, ganlion cyst (e.g. temporomandibular, wrist, elbow or ankle, aromioclavicular, olecranon bursa)	38.08	3	80.30	88.00	78.10
20610	Arthrocentesis, aspiration and/or injection; major joint or bursa (e.g. shoulder, hip, knee, joint, subacrominal bursa)	41.68	3	93.50	102.30	91.30
62270	Spinal puncture, lumbar, diagnositc	61.39	5	172.70	178.20	169.40
62273	Injection, lumbar epidural of blood or clot patch	113.78	8	414.70	427.90	408.10
62274	Injection of anesthestic substance, (including narcotics) diagnostic or therapeutic, subarachnoid or subdural, single	86.86	8	388.30	401.50	382.80
62275	Injection of anesthestic substance, (including narcotics) diagnostic or therapeutic, epidural, cervical or thoracic single	82.99	10	492.80	508.20	485.10
62276	Injection of anesthestic substance, (including narcotics) diagnostic or therapeutic, subarachnoid or subdural, differential	112.80	8	414.70	427.90	408.10
62277	Injection of anesthestic substance, (including narcotics) diagnostic or therapeutic, subarachnoid or subdural, continuous	103.97	8	414.70	427.90	408.10
62278	Injection of anesthestic substance, (including narcotics) diagnostic or therapeutic, epidural, lumbar, or caudal single	88.40	8	427.90	441.10	421.30
62279	Epidural, lumbar, or caudal, continuous (not to include continous analgesia for labor and vaginal delivery or caesarean section)	84.97	8	569.80	588.50	561.00
62280	Injection of neurolytic substance, (e.g. alcohol, phenol, iced saline solutions); subarachnoid	112.78	20	388.30	401.50	382.80
62281	Injection of neurolytic substance, (e.g. alcohol, phenol, iced saline solutions); epidural, cervical, or thoracic	123.05	22	492.80	508.20	485.10
62282	Injection of neurolytic substance, (e.g. alcohol, phenol, iced saline solutions); epidural, lumbar, or caudal	142.37	20	518.10	534.60	510.40
62288	Injection of substance other than anesthetic, contrast, or neurolytic, subarachnoid (seperate procedure)	99.79	8	388.30	401.50	382.80
62289	Injection of substance other than anesthetic, contrast, or neurolytic, lumbar or caudal (seperate procedure)	96.41	8	427.90	441.10	421.30
62298	Injection of substance other than anesthetic, contrast, or neurolytic, epidural, cervical or thoracic (seperate procedure)	108.98	10	492.80	508.20	485.10
62350	Implantation, revision or repositioning of intrathecal or epidural catheter, for implantable reservoir or implantable infusion pump; without laminectomy	366.36	26	2,850.10	2,942.50	2,807.20
62355	Removal of previously implanted intrathecal or epidural catheter	309.84	18	1,295.80	1,337.60	1,276.00
62360	Implantation or replacement of device for intathecal or epidural drug infusion; subcutaneous reservoir	131.22	16	1,347.50	1,391.50	1,326.60
62361	Implantation or replacement of device for intathecal or epidural drug infusion; non-programmable pump	285.96	19	1,347.50	1,391.50	1,326.60
62362	Implantation or replacement of device for intathecal or epidural drug infusion; programmable pump, including preparation of pump, with or without programming	372.56	25	1,424.50	1,471.80	1,403.60
62365	Removal of subcutaneous reserviour or pump, previously implanted for intathecal or epidural infusion	308.22	16	854.70	883.30	842.60

Medicare allowable from *Kentucky Medicare Part B 1998 Participation Program for Physicians with Participation 1998 Physician Fee Schedule*. ASA Relative Value from American Society of Anesthesiologists *1998 Relative Value Guide: A Guide for Anesthesia Values*, Park Ridge, Illinois.

75% Avg. Physician Charge	95% Avg. Physician Charge	50% Avg. Physician/ASA Rel. Value	75% Avg. Physician/ASA Rel. Value	Proposed Fee	Proposed Fee/ASA Rel. Value	Proposed Fee/50% Avg. Physician	Proposed Fee/75% Avg. Physician
86.90	119.90	26.03	28.97	150.00	50.00	1.92	1.73
80.30	110.00	23.83	26.77	150.00	50.00	2.10	1.87
86.90	119.90	26.03	28.97	150.00	50.00	1.92	1.73
102.30	140.80	30.43	34.10	150.00	50.00	1.64	1.47
177.10	191.40	33.88	35.42	250.00	50.00	1.48	1.41
426.80	460.90	51.01	53.35	400.00	50.00	0.98	0.94
400.40	431.20	47.85	50.05	400.00	50.00	1.04	1.00
507.10	546.70	48.51	50.71	500.00	50.00	1.03	0.99
426.80	460.90	51.01	53.35	400.00	50.00	0.98	0.94
426.80	460.90	51.01	53.35	400.00	50.00	0.98	0.94
440.00	475.20	52.66	55.00	400.00	50.00	0.95	0.91
587.40	632.50	70.13	73.42	400.00	50.00	0.71	0.68
400.40	431.20	19.14	20.02	1,000.00	50.00	2.61	2.50
507.10	546.70	22.05	23.05	1,100.00	50.00	2.27	2.17
533.50	575.30	25.52	26.67	1,000.00	50.00	1.96	1.87
400.40	431.20	47.85	50.05	400.00	50.00	1.04	1.00
440.00	475.20	52.66	55.00	400.00	50.00	0.95	0.91
507.10	546.70	48.51	50.71	500.00	50.00	1.03	0.99
2,934.80	3,164.70	107.97	112.88	1,300.00	50.00	0.46	0.44
1,334.30	1,438.80	70.89	74.13	900.00	50.00	0.71	0.67
1,387.10	1,496.00	82.91	86.69	800.00	50.00	0.60	0.58
1,387.10	1,496.00	69.82	73.01	950.00	50.00	0.72	0.68
1,467.40	1,582.90	56.14	58.70	1,250.00	50.00	0.89	0.85
880.00	949.30	52.66	55.00	800.00	50.00	0.95	0.91

Average Indemnity Insurance Low and High, 50%, 75%, 95% physician charge were created for this example and are not based upon actual data from any source.

jections, SI joint injections, and spinal puncture have ratios that are greater than one. While more complex procedures such as implantation of an epidural catheter and removal of previously implanted epidural catheter have ratios that are less than one. This would indicate that most physicians charge less per ASA relative value unit for less complex procedures and more for more complex procedures.

This pricing approach is based upon the relative value of the procedures that you perform and does not take into consideration the costs of providing those services.

- **Cost Plus Pricing Method.** Forecast the cost of providing the service by estimating the direct costs by procedure, allocating a charge per procedure for overhead (indirect expenses), and then adding a mark-up for profit. To determine overhead by procedure, estimate the overhead for the practice for the year. Forecast the frequency (number of procedures) by CPT-4 code that will be performed in the year. Multiple the ASA relative value times the frequency to determine the total relative value units that your practice will be providing. Divide the total overhead for the year by the total relative value units to determine a cost per unit. Then, multiply the cost per unit by the number of units per procedure to determine the overhead allocation per procedure. The total mark-up for the practice is usually established as a single number, which is equal to the estimated annual income for all the physicians in the group divided by the total ASA relative value units. This determines the markup per procedure *(see Figure 2)*.

This pricing approach is based upon recovering direct and overhead costs and generating a profit, but it also relies heavily upon your ability to forecast the number of procedures that you will perform. If the forecast is inaccurate, overhead will be over- or under-absorbed which will result in increased profitability or loss.

This approach is also helpful when analyzing managed care contracts. Assuming that overhead is fixed, if the proposed reimbursement from the managed care contract drops below the

FIGURE 2: COST PLUS PRICING (Partial List)

CPT-4	CPT-4 Code Description	1988 Frequency	ASA Relative Value	ASA Relative Value Frequency	Direct Cost per CPT-4 Code	Overhead Cost Per CPT-4 Code	Mark-up	Proposed Fee
20550	Injection, tendon sheath, ligament, trigger points, or ganglion cyst	1,267	3	3,801	3.67	32.88	22.80	59.34
20600	Arthrocentesis, aspiration and/or injection; small joint, bursa or ganlion cyst (e.g. fingers, toes)	34	3	102	3.67	32.88	22.80	59.34
20605	Arthrocentesis, aspiration and/or injection; intermediate joint, bursa, ganlion cyst (e.g. temporomandibular, wrist, elbow or ankle, aromioclavicular, olecranon bursa)	115	3	345	3.67	32.88	22.80	59.34
20610	Arthrocentesis, aspiration and/or injection; major joint or bursa (e.g. shoulder, hip, knee, joint, subacrominal bursa)	959	3	2,877	3.67	32.88	22.80	59.34
62270	Spinal puncture, lumbar, diagnositc	4	5	20	n/a	54.79	38.00	92.79
62273	Injection, lumbar epidural of blood or clot patch	23	8	184	n/a	87.67	60.79	148.46
62274	Injection of anesthetic substance, (including narcotics) diagnostic or therapeutic, subarachnoid or subdural, single	0	8	0	n/a	87.67	60.79	148.46
62275	Injection of anesthetic substance, (including narcotics) diagnostic or therapeutic, epidural, cervical or thoracic single	224	10	2,240	n/a	109.58	75.99	185.58
62276	Injection of anesthetic substance, (including narcotics) diagnostic or therapeutic, subarachnoid or subdural, differential	0	8	0	n/a	87.67	60.79	148.46
62277	Injection of anesthetic substance, (including narcotics) diagnostic or therapeutic, subarachnoid or subdural, continuous	0	8	0	n/a	87.67	60.79	148.46
62278	Injection of anesthetic substance, (including narcotics) diagnostic or therapeutic, epidural, lumbar, or caudal single	1,131	8	9,048	n/a	87.67	60.79	148.46
62279	Epidural, lumbar, or caudal, continuous (not to include continous analgesia for labor and vaginal delivery or caesarean section)	37	8	296	n/a	87.67	60.79	148.46
62280	Injection of neurolytic substance, (e.g. alcohol, phenol, iced saline solutions); subarachnoid	0	20	0	n/a	219.17	151.99	371.15
62281	Injection of neurolytic substance, (e.g. alcohol, phenol, iced saline solutions); epidural, cervical, or thoracic	0	22	0	n/a	241.08	167.18	408.27
62282	Injection of neurolytic substance, (e.g. alcohol, phenol, iced saline solutions); epidural, lumbar, or caudal	0	20	0	n/a	219.17	151.99	371.15
62288	Injection of substance other than anesthetic, contrast, or neurolytic, subarachnoid (seperate procedure)	11	8	88	n/a	87.67	60.79	148.46
62289	Injection of substance other than anesthetic, contrast, or neurolytic, lumbar or caudal (seperate procedure)	1,503	8	12,024	n/a	87.67	60.79	148.46
62298	Injection of substance other than anesthetic, contrast, or neurolytic, epidural, cervical or thoracic (seperate procedure)	816	10	8,160	n/a	109.58	75.99	185.58
62350	Implantation, revision or repositioning of intrathecal or epidural catheter, for implantable reservoir or implantable infusion pump; without laminectomy	10	26	260	n/a	284.92	197.58	482.50
62355	Removal of previously implanted intrathecal or epidural catheter	2	18	36	n/a	197.25	136.79	334.04
62360	Implantation or replacement of device for intrathecal or epidural drug infusion; subcutaneous reservoir	6	16	96	n/a	175.33	121.59	296.92
62361	Implantation or replacement of device for intrathecal or epidural drug infusion; non-programmable pump	3	19	57	n/a	208.21	144.39	352.60
62362	Implantation or replacement of device for intrathecal or epidural drug infusion; programmable pump, including preparation of pump, with or without programming	8	25	200	n/a	273.96	189.98	463.94
62365	Removal of subcutaneous reserviour or pump, previously implanted for intrathecal or epidural infusion	5	16	80	n/a	175.33	121.59	296.92
**	**	*	*	*	*	*	*	*
	TOTAL	12,993		84,219				

ASA Relative Value from American Society of Anesthesiologists, *1998 Relative Value Guide: A Guide for Anesthesia Values*, Park Ridge, Illinois.
Overhead cost per CPT-4 code has a "n/a" or not applicable in the column if the procedure is performed at a hospital or surgery center because they will be reimbursed for the supplies utilized.

FIGURE 2: COST PLUS PRICING (Continued)

Overhead Cost per ASA Relative Value Unit = Estimated Annual Overhead/Total ASA Relative Value Units

Overhead Cost per CPT-4 Code = Cost per ASA Relative Value Unit x ASA Relative Value Units

Estimated Annual Overhead   922,900
Total ASA Relative Value Units   84,219

Cost per ASA Relative Value Unit   922,900/84,219 =10.96

Markup per ASA Relative Value Unit = Estimated Annual Physicians Salary/Total ASA Relative Value Units

Markup per CPT-4 Code = ASA Relative Value Unit x ASA Relative Value Units

Estimated Annual Physicians Salary   640,000 (two physicians at $320,000 each per year)
Total ASA Relative Value Units   84,219

Markup Per Relative Value Unit =   640,000/84,219 = 7.60

---

proposed, fee then the physicians' income will be decreased. Conversely, if the reimbursement from the managed care contract is greater than the proposed fee, then the physicians' income will be increased.

- **Marketplace Average Method.** Average the 50th and 75th percentile of what most physicians' charge according to the *Physician Fee Analyzer Plus* or similar book. This method is based upon the economic theory of supply and demand: when a practice enters into a market with many competitors, then the average or near average price has already been established *(see Figure 3)*. Notice that the numbers in the last two columns are almost equal to one, indicating the proposed fee is close to what other physicians are charging. Like the ASA relative value method, this approach does not take into consideration the costs involved in providing those services.

Finalize Fee Schedule

Once you have completed the spreadsheets, analyze the data. Ask the following questions:
- Are the proposed fees reasonable?

Pricing — Creating a Fee Schedule

- Are the proposed fees above or equal to the 50th percentile, but below or equal to the 75th percentile of what other physicians charge?
- Are the proposed fees within the range of what most insurance companies will reimburse?
- Can you in good conscience defend the fees as reasonable?
- Can you earn a reasonable profit if you were paid at this fee level? Profit is equal to income minus expenses. Income is based upon negotiated reimbursement and not the fee charges listed on the fee schedule.

As a general rule, fees that are too high could jeopardize your ability to obtain managed care contracts. High fees can create an image for your patients, referring physicians, and others in the community that you are greedy. Conversely, fees that are too low could jeopardize your income. Low fees can also create the perception of poor quality.

The purpose of analyzing the data is to perform a reasonableness check. Notice that a proposed fee can vary widely depending upon the method. For example, a trigger point injection was priced at $150.00 *(Relative Value Method, Figure 1)*, $59.34 *(Cost Plus Pricing Method, Figure 2)*, and $82.50 *(Market Place Average Method, Figure 3)* respectively. The Medicare allowable for a trigger point injection is $41.43, $17.91 below the Cost Plus Pricing method of providing the service. If the practice provides trigger point injections to Medicare patients, they will do so at a loss. Further note that the mark-up for this procedure is $22.80, thus the loss will result in lower income to the physicians. After analyzing the data from all three approaches, determine a reasonable fair market value proposed fee *(see Figure 4)*.

FIGURE 3: MARKETPLACE AVERAGE METHOD (partial list)

CPT-4 Code	CPT-4 Code Description	Medicare Allowable	ASA Relative Value	Average Indemnity Low	Average Indemnity High	50% Avg. Physician Charge
20550	Injection, tendon sheath, ligament, trigger points, or ganglion cyst	41.43	3	80.30	88.00	78.10
20600	Arthrocentesis, aspiration and/or injection; small joint, bursa or ganlion cyst (e.g. fingers, toes)	38.07	3	73.70	80.30	71.50
20605	Arthrocentesis, aspiration and/or injection; intermediate joint, bursa, ganlion cyst (e.g. temporomandibular, wrist, elbow or ankle, aromioclavicular, olecranon bursa)	38.08	3	80.30	88.00	78.10
20610	Arthrocentesis, aspiration and/or injection; major joint or bursa (e.g. shoulder, hip, knee, joint, subacrominal bursa)	41.68	3	93.50	102.30	91.30
62270	Spinal puncture, lumbar, diagnositc	61.39	5	172.70	178.20	169.40
62273	Injection, lumbar epidural of blood or clot patch	113.78	8	414.70	427.90	408.10
62274	Injection of anesthestic substance, (including narcotics) diagnostic or therapeutic, subarachnoid or subdural, single	86.86	8	388.30	401.50	382.80
62275	Injection of anesthestic substance, (including narcotics) diagnostic or therapeutic, epidural, cervical or thoracic single	82.99	10	492.80	508.20	485.10
62276	Injection of anesthestic substance, (including narcotics) diagnostic or therapeutic, subarachnoid or subdural, differential	112.80	8	414.70	427.90	408.10
62277	Injection of anesthestic substance, (including narcotics) diagnostic or therapeutic, subarachnoid or subdural, continuous	103.97	8	414.70	427.90	408.10
62278	Injection of anesthestic substance, (including narcotics) diagnostic or therapeutic, epidural, lumbar, or caudal single	88.40	8	427.90	441.10	421.30
62279	Epidural, lumbar, or caudal, continuous (not to include continous analgesia for labor and vaginal delivery or caesarean section)	84.97	8	569.80	588.50	561.00
62280	Injection of neurolytic substance, (e.g. alcohol, phenol, iced saline solutions); subarachnoid	112.78	20	388.30	401.50	382.80
62281	Injection of neurolytic substance, (e.g. alcohol, phenol, iced saline solutions); epidural, cervical, or thoracic	123.05	22	492.80	508.20	485.10
62282	Injection of neurolytic substance, (e.g. alcohol, phenol, iced saline solutions); epidural, lumbar, or caudal	142.37	20	518.10	534.60	510.40
62288	Injection of substance other than anesthetic, contrast, or neurolytic, subarachnoid (seperate procedure)	99.79	8	388.30	401.50	382.80
62289	Injection of substance other than anesthetic, contrast, or neurolytic, lumbar or caudal (seperate procedure)	96.41	8	427.90	441.10	421.30
62298	Injection of substance other than anesthetic, contrast, or neurolytic, epidural, cervical or thoracic (seperate procedure)	108.98	10	492.80	508.20	485.10
62350	Implantation, revision or repositioning of intrathecal or epidural catheter, for implantable reservoir or implantable infusion pump; without laminectomy	366.36	26	2,850.10	2,942.50	2,807.20
62355	Removal of previously implanted intrathecal or epidural catheter	309.84	18	1,295.80	1,337.60	1,276.00
62360	Implantation or replacement of device for intathecal or epidural drug infusion; subcutaneous reservoir	131.22	16	1,347.50	1,391.50	1,326.60
62361	Implantation or replacement of device for intathecal or epidural drug infusion; non-programmable pump	285.96	19	1,347.50	1,391.50	1,326.60
62362	Implantation or replacement of device for intathecal or epidural drug infusion; programmable pump, including preparation of pump, with or without programming	372.56	25	1,424.50	1,471.80	1,403.60
62365	Removal of subcutaneous reserviour or pump, previously implanted for intathecal or epidural infusion	308.22	16	854.70	883.30	842.60

Medicare allowable from *Kentucky Medicare Part B 1998 Participation Program for Physicians with Participation 1998 Physician Fee Schedule.* ASA Relative Value from American Society of Anesthesiologists *1998 Relative Value Guide: A Guide for Anesthesia Values,* Park Ridge, Illinois.

75% Avg. Physician Charge	95% Avg. Physician Charge	50% Avg. Physician/ASA Rel. Value	75% Avg. Physician/ASA Rel. Value	Proposed Fee	Proposed Fee/ASA Rel. Value	Proposed Fee/50% Avg. Physician	Proposed Fee/75% Avg. Physician
86.90	119.90	26.03	28.97	82.50	27.50	1.06	0.95
80.30	110.00	23.83	26.77	75.90	25.30	1.06	0.95
86.90	119.90	26.03	28.97	82.50	27.50	1.06	0.95
102.30	140.80	30.43	34.10	96.80	32.27	1.06	0.95
177.10	191.40	33.88	35.42	173.25	34.65	1.02	0.98
426.80	460.90	51.01	53.35	417.45	52.18	1.02	0.98
400.40	431.20	47.85	50.05	391.60	48.95	1.02	0.98
507.10	546.70	48.51	50.71	496.10	49.61	1.02	0.98
426.80	460.90	51.01	53.35	417.45	52.18	1.02	0.98
426.80	460.90	51.01	53.35	417.45	52.18	1.02	0.98
440.00	475.20	52.66	55.00	430.65	53.83	1.02	0.98
587.40	632.50	70.13	73.42	574.20	71.78	1.02	0.98
400.40	431.20	19.14	20.02	391.60	19.58	1.02	0.98
507.10	546.70	22.05	23.05	496.10	22.55	1.02	0.98
533.50	575.30	25.52	26.67	521.95	26.10	1.02	0.98
400.40	431.20	47.85	50.05	391.60	48.95	1.02	0.98
440.00	475.20	52.66	55.00	430.65	53.83	1.02	0.98
507.10	546.70	48.51	50.71	496.10	49.61	1.02	0.98
2,934.80	3,164.70	107.97	112.88	2,871.00	110.42	1.02	0.98
1,334.30	1,438.80	70.89	74.13	1,305.15	72.51	1.02	0.98
1,387.10	1,496.00	82.91	86.69	1,356.85	84.80	1.02	0.98
1,387.10	1,496.00	69.82	73.01	1,356.85	71.41	1.02	0.98
1,467.40	1,582.90	56.14	58.70	1,435.50	57.42	1.02	0.98
880.00	949.30	52.66	55.00	861.30	53.83	1.02	0.98

Average Indemnity Insurance Low and High, 50%, 75%, 95% physician charge were created for this example and are not based upon actual data from any source.

FIGURE 4: ANALYSIS OF ALL METHODS

CPT-4 Code	CPT-4 Code Description	Medicare Allowable	ASA Relative Value	Average Indemnity Low	Average Indemnity High	50% Avg. Physician Charge
20550	Injection, tendon sheath, ligament, trigger points, or ganglion cyst	41.43	3	80.30	88.00	78.10
20600	Arthrocentesis, aspiration and/or injection; small joint, bursa or ganlion cyst (e.g. fingers, toes)	38.07	3	73.70	80.30	71.50
20605	Arthrocentesis, aspiration and/or injection; intermediate joint, bursa, ganlion cyst (e.g. temporomandibular, wrist, elbow or ankle, aromioclavicular, olecranon bursa)	38.08	3	80.30	88.00	78.10
20610	Arthrocentesis, aspiration and/or injection; major joint or bursa (e.g. shoulder, hip, knee, joint, subacrominal bursa)	41.68	3	93.50	102.30	91.30
62270	Spinal puncture, lumbar, diagnositc	61.39	5	172.70	178.20	169.40
62273	Injection, lumbar epidural of blood or clot patch	113.78	8	414.70	427.90	408.10
62274	Injection of anesthestic substance, (including narcotics) diagnostic or therapeutic, subarachnoid or subdural, single	86.86	8	388.30	401.50	382.80
62275	Injection of anesthestic substance, (including narcotics) diagnostic or therapeutic, epidural, cervical or thoracic single	82.99	10	492.80	508.20	485.10
62276	Injection of anesthestic substance, (including narcotics) diagnostic or therapeutic, subarachnoid or subdural, differential	112.80	8	414.70	427.90	408.10
62277	Injection of anesthestic substance, (including narcotics) diagnostic or therapeutic, subarachnoid or subdural, continuous	103.97	8	414.70	427.90	408.10
62278	Injection of anesthestic substance, (including narcotics) diagnostic or therapeutic, epidural, lumbar, or caudal single	88.40	8	427.90	441.10	421.30
62279	Epidural, lumbar, or caudal, continuous (not to include continous analgesia for labor and vaginal delivery or caesarean section)	84.97	8	569.80	588.50	561.00
62280	Injection of neurolytic substance, (e.g. alcohol, phenol, iced saline solutions); subarachnoid	112.78	20	388.30	401.50	382.80
62281	Injection of neurolytic substance, (e.g. alcohol, phenol, iced saline solutions); epidural, cervical, or thoracic	123.05	22	492.80	508.20	485.10
62282	Injection of neurolytic substance, (e.g. alcohol, phenol, iced saline solutions); epidural, lumbar, or caudal	142.37	20	518.10	534.60	510.40
62288	Injection of substance other than anesthetic, contrast, or neurolytic, subarachnoid (seperate procedure)	99.79	8	388.30	401.50	382.80
62289	Injection of substance other than anesthetic, contrast, or neurolytic, lumbar or caudal (seperate procedure)	96.41	8	427.90	441.10	421.30
62298	Injection of substance other than anesthetic, contrast, or neurolytic, epidural, cervical or thoracic (seperate procedure)	108.98	10	492.80	508.20	485.10
62350	Implantation, revision or repositioning of intrathecal or epidural catheter, for implantable reservoir or implantable infusion pump; without laminectomy	366.36	26	2,850.10	2,942.50	2,807.20
62355	Removal of previously implanted intrathecal or epidural catheter	309.84	18	1,295.80	1,337.60	1,276.00
62360	Implantation or replacement of device for intathecal or epidural drug infusion; subcutaneous reservoir	131.22	16	1,347.50	1,391.50	1,326.60
62361	Implantation or replacement of device for intathecal or epidural drug infusion; non-programmable pump	285.96	19	1,347.50	1,391.50	1,326.60
62362	Implantation or replacement of device for intathecal or epidural drug infusion; programmable pump, including preparation of pump, with or without programming	372.56	25	1,424.50	1,471.80	1,403.60
62365	Removal of subcutaneous reserviour or pump, previously implanted for intathecal or epidural infusion	308.22	16	854.70	883.30	842.60

Medicare allowable from Kentucky Medicare Part B 1998 Participation Program for Physicians with Participation 1998 Physician Fee Schedule. ASA Relative Value from American Society of Anesthesiologists *1998 Relative Value Guide: A Guide for Anesthesia Values,* Park Ridge, Illinois.

	75% Avg. Physician Charge	95% Avg. Physician Charge	ASA Relative Value Method	Cost Plus Pricing Method	Marketplace Average Method	Proposed Fee
			\multicolumn{3}{c}{PROPOSED FEE}	
	86.90	119.90	150.00	59.34	82.50	85.00
	80.30	110.00	150.00	59.34	75.90	85.00
	86.90	119.90	150.00	59.34	82.50	85.00
	102.30	140.80	150.00	59.34	96.80	100.00
	177.10	191.40	250.00	92.79	173.25	175.00
	426.80	460.90	400.00	148.46	417.45	425.00
	400.40	431.20	400.00	148.46	391.60	400.00
	507.10	546.70	500.00	185.58	496.10	500.00
	426.80	460.90	400.00	148.46	417.45	425.00
	426.80	460.90	400.00	148.46	417.45	425.00
	440.00	475.20	400.00	148.46	430.65	435.00
	587.40	632.50	400.00	148.46	574.20	600.00
	400.40	431.20	1,000.00	371.15	391.60	400.00
	507.10	546.70	1,100.00	408.27	496.10	500.00
	533.50	575.30	1,000.00	371.15	521.95	525.00
	400.40	431.20	400.00	148.46	391.60	400.00
	440.00	475.20	400.00	148.46	430.65	430.00
	507.10	546.70	500.00	185.58	496.10	500.00
	2,934.80	3,164.70	1,300.00	482.50	2,871.00	2,875.00
	1,334.30	1,438.80	900.00	334.04	1,305.15	1,300.00
	1,387.10	1,496.00	800.00	296.92	1,356.85	1,350.00
	1,387.10	1,496.00	950.00	352.60	1,356.85	1,350.00
	1,467.40	1,582.90	1,250.00	453.94	1,435.50	1,450.00
	880.00	949.30	800.00	296.92	861.30	875.00

Average Indemnity Insurance Low and High, 50%, 75%, 95% physician charge were created for this example and are not based upon actual data from any source.

CHAPTER 6
Practice Name, Image, and Goodwill

"It takes twenty years to build a reputation and five minutes to ruin it."
–Warren Buffet

"As long as you are going to think anyway, think big."
–Donald Trump

An image is a complete package that embodies the essence of the practice. You are building a practice and someday you will likely retire and sell your practice either to your partners or to an investor. If you create your image correctly, you can build a practice that has "goodwill." Goodwill is an accounting term that is used to describe intangible assets associated with a practice. When a practice is an on-going operation, there is no calculation or accounting for goodwill; however, when a practice is sold, goodwill is the amount that the purchaser is willing to pay for a business in excess of the sum of its assets minus its liabilities. The purchaser will pay more for an on-going practice that has intangible assets such as an established patient base, patient loyalty, referring physicians' loyalty, and image. *The greater the goodwill the more the practice is worth.*

Establishing an image that builds goodwill begins with the creation of your name, logo, design and color choices, and position statement. Goodwill grows as you promote your image while meeting your target markets' needs and wants.

What is the image that you think of when you think of a Coca-Cola®? Can you see the trademarked bottle and logo of "The Real Thing™"? Every time that you see the Coke® logo it is printed in the unmistakable Coca-Cola® red. A tremendous amount of effort and money has gone into the promotion of Coke®. How much do you think The Coca-Cola® Company would be willing to sell their logo for? The logo's only value is in the goodwill that is associated with its image.

What are the images that you think of when you think of The Mayo Clinic, The Cleveland Clinic, and John-Hopkins Medical Center? These centers have created a national reputation of excellence. Patients with complicated medical problems are referred to these institutions because they have a reputation for diagnosing and treating rare and/or difficult cases using the most current technological advances available in medicine.

Naming the Practice

Developing the image of your practice starts with creating a name. The decision of what to name your practice should be well thought out. Names can describe what you do, who you are, and/or where you are located. For example, a practice can be named based upon what you do, such as Pain Management Associates or The Pain Clinic. Names can be based upon what you do and where you are located, as in Midwest Pain Associates, or The Chicago Pain Institute. A practice can also be named using the partners' names, such as Smith and Jones, or Dickinson, Stewart and Vanderberg.

Practices named for what they do can quickly establish goodwill. Descriptive and geographical names need to be specific, but not too narrow nor too broad. A name such as Midwest Pain Center, or Southeast Pain Anesthesiology Associates, are broader and less limiting than a name like East Louisville Pain Clinic or South Kansas City Pain Management Associates.

Naming your practice after large cities such as Chicago or Philadelphia is less limiting than naming your practice after smaller cities like Allentown or Springfield. If you are in a smaller city and want to expand to a neighboring city, the neighboring city's target markets may be offended that you are using the base city's name. For example, let's assume that there are two small cities, one named Corbin and the other named Barbourville. You locate your practice in Corbin and name it the Corbin Pain Associates. You decide to expand to Barbourville, and you keep the Corbin Pain Associates name. The people in Barbourville may feel that you are not part of their community solely on account of the name. If you had named your practice Southeastern Kentucky Pain Associates, neither community would be offended.

Practices that use the partners' last names must decide if they will change the name of the practice when they add additional partners or if original partners leave the practice. Changing the name of a practice can decrease goodwill and cause confusion in the market. Practices can continue to use their original name even though they have added new partners and some partners have retired. If a group has been practicing in a community for some time and has already established a reputation for excellence, then using the names of the partners may provide instant goodwill.

Once a name has been selected, it must be researched to make sure that the name is unique and available. To find out, seek the expertise of an attorney who specializes in intellectual property (trademarks, servicemarks, and copyrights). Ask him/her to research the proposed practice name in your state to see if the name that you have selected is in use or is reserved for use by someone else. Depending upon how geographically broad you want to be, you may also want to perform a national search to see if anyone is using this name nationally. If the name is in use, you will need to select another name.

The Logo Design and Color Choice

The image you project includes your name, your logo, choice of colors, and position statement. A logo design and its colors

Practice Name, Image, and Goodwill

are an artistic representation of your image, and as the old adage states, a picture can say a thousand words. Think about the feeling that you want to convey. What colors do you like? Have you always liked these colors? Are these colors trendy and likely to become dated? In the medical community, most physicians use either shades of blue or green.

You may choose to use the same colors that others are using, or you may want to be different. Red is rarely used in the medical community because it is signifies an allergy, an emergency, and blood. Most logos are two colors, but they can be up to four colors (note that all colors can be created with four-color processing). The more colors used, the more your printing costs will escalate. The colors that you choose for your logo become a part of your corporate image and should remain consistent in all marketing literature that you create. Just as the Coca-Cola® logo is always in an unmistakable red color, your logo should also use a consistent color scheme.

Once you have decided on the feeling and colors that you like, you can seek the help of a qualified graphic artist who specializes in business logo and trademark development. If you like samples of his/her work, ask the graphic artist to prepare several ideas for a logo for your practice. Discuss with the graphic artist the feelings you want to convey and the colors that you like, but also listen to his/her advice. It often takes several iterations to develop the logo design.

The Position Statement

While you are developing the logo, think about your position statement. A position statement can be thought of a slogan. Coke® uses the slogan "The Real Thing™." The combination of the practice's name, logo design, color choice, and position statement creates your image. Examples of position statements are:
- Dedicated to the treatment of acute and chronic pain.
- Dedicated to relieving your pain.
- Providing excellence in pain management.
- The source for back pain treatment.

The Keys to Successful Marketing

- Dedicated to patient-friendly pain relief.
- Specializing in cancer pain management.

Once you have decided on the name, logo, colors, and position statement, ask your attorney to file for a servicemark. A **servicemark** legally protects intellectual property of a business that provides a service. A **trademark** legally protects intellectual property of a business that produces a product.

CHAPTER 7
Choosing a Legal Entity

"A traveller without knowledge is a bird without wings."
–Sa' Di Gulistan

Your attorney and accountant can advise and assist you in establishing the legal entity for your practice. There are many legal entities, including proprietorship, partnership, limited liability partnership, C corporation, sub-chapter S corporation, non-profit organization, and limited liability company. Most medical practices are incorporated as a sub-chapter S corporation. This legal entity is also referred to as a professional services corporation (PSC). However, a new entity called a limited liability company (LLC) is gaining in popularity. These various options have different tax and liability consequences. It is important to realize that no matter what type of legal structure you choose, a physician can not use a legal structure to reduce his/her medical malpractice liability.

Sole Proprietorship

A sole proprietorship is owned by one individual who has no liability protection under the law for business debt or litigation. Sole proprietorships are taxed at an individual level and cease to exist upon the death of the individual who created them. When a sole proprietor commits the business to a contract, she/he is also committing to be personally liable for the commitments made in the contract.

Partnership

A partnership is a voluntary relationship that is formed when two or more people agree, usually in writing, to pool resources to form a partnership, that is a for-profit business entity with more than one owner, which ceases upon death, bankruptcy, or termination of the agreement by any partner. Every partner can legally bind the partnership to any contract. And, all partners are personally liable for debts or negligent acts incurred by the partnership.

Proceeds from a partnership flow through to the owner's individual income tax returns, whether or not they are distributed to the individuals. Partnerships also pass losses through to the individual partners, thus making them an excellent legal entity structure for the ownership of real estate. Proceeds and losses of the partnership can flow through to the partners based upon their basis, the amount each partner has invested in the partnership. For example, if one partner has invested five times as much as another partner, the law views that it is only fair that this be taken into consideration when distributing income.

Limited Liability Partnership

A limited liability partnership is similar to a partnership except limited partners cannot have a role in management of the partnership and are limited in their liability to the amount that they have invested in the partnership.

C Corporation

A C corporation is a legal entity that is separate and distinct from its owners and therefore is provided with liability

Choosing a Legal Entity

protection for its owners who are referred to as shareholders or stockholders. Most large corporations in the United States are organized as C corporations. A corporation can establish different classes of stock such as common stock and preferred stock, which have different voting rights. In 1819, Chief Justice John Marshall defined a corporation as "an artificial being, invisible, intangible, and existing only in the contemplation of the law." A corporation is considered a separate legal entity and by law is granted all rights and responsibilities as an individual except the right to vote and marry. A corporation can sue and be sued; buy, sell, and own property; and enter into contracts.

A corporation has an unlimited life, continuing after the death of its shareholders. Shareholders own stock in the corporation that they can sell at will. Shareholders are not liable for actions of the corporation or the debts incurred by the corporation. Each shareholder has the right to vote to make decisions about the corporation's future one vote for each share of stock owned. A shareholder does not have the right to bind the corporation to any contract.

Corporations, except for certain federal charters granted to banks and saving and loans, are governed by the laws of the state in which they were incorporated. A corporation is established by creating the charter or articles of incorporation. This document, which varies from state to state, usually specifies the corporation's name, business purpose, address, amount of stock issued, par value of the stock, number of directors, and the names, address and number of shares owned by each director. The corporation is governed by the by-laws, a document which specifies the internal management of the corporation, such as how many directors are to be elected, how the directors are elected, provisions for issuing stock, number and type of management committees, and the duties of each committee.

Corporations pay corporate income tax on earnings at a rate that is lower than individual rates. When proceeds are distributed to shareholders in the form of dividends, the shareholder is taxed at individual tax rates. This is often referred to as double-taxation of dividends. Losses of a corporation do not flow through to its owners; thus losses get trapped in the corporation and cannot provide a tax benefit to the shareholders. For this reason a C corporation is usually not the best choice of entity for holding real estate.

Sub-Chapter S Corporation

A sub-chapter S corporation, or professional services corporation (PSC), is a highbred which combines the attributes of both the partnership and corporation together. A sub-charter S corporation is established and governed like a C corporation and taxed like a partnership. Most physician-established sub-chapter S corporations specify in their charter that shareholders must be licensed physicians, and how, when, and at what price stock ownership is transferred or sold to new shareholders. Like a C corporation, shareholders of a sub-chapter S corporation cannot obligate the corporation to a contract, and shareholders are provided with liability protection for the debts, acts of negligence, and contractual agreements of the corporation. However, unlike a C corporation, sub-chapter S corporations can only have one class of stock, and each share of stock must have the same rights and dividends. Like a partnership, income and losses of the corporation flow through to the shareholders. However, unlike a partnership, sub-chapter S corporations cannot include their share of the losses in their basis.

Non-Profit Organizations

Internal Revenue Code 501(c)(3) is used to grant non-profit organizations exemptions from federal income tax for those who qualify based upon educational, religious, or charitable purposes. Tax exemptions are also granted to organizations that serve the public interest and are owned by a city, state, or local government entity. To qualify for tax exemption, the organization must prove that:
- It benefits the public interest.
- It is granted the exemption from the Internal Revenue Service.

Choosing a Legal Entity

- It ensures that its shareholders, or individual directors, defined as anyone who has control or influence over the organization's operations, receive no part of the net earnings of the organization.

The Internal Revenue Service scrutinizes non-profit tax-exempt entities very closely, including physician-hospital affiliations. Most physician practices do not qualify for non-profit tax status.

Limited Liability Company

A limited liability company (LLC) is another hybrid legal structure which provides limited liability to its partners, is governed like a corporation, taxed like a partnership, and provides for free transferability of interest.

Ask your attorney and accountant for advice on the best type of legal entity for your practice.

EXAMPLE
Steps to Set Up a Sub-Chapter S Corporation

For example, let's assume that your practice will be established as a sub-chapter S corporation. Your attorney will create the by-laws, stock certificates, and articles of incorporation which will be filed in the state in which you want to incorporate. Once incorporated, your accountant can assist in filing forms to request a federal tax ID and sub-chapter S election. Your practice will be incorporated in only one state, but you can still practice in other states.

CHAPTER 8
Advertising and Selling

*"If you think that advertising doesn't pay —
we understand that there are twenty-five mountains
in Colorado higher than Pike's Peak. Can you name one?"*
–The American Salesman

"To be in hell is to drift, to be in heaven is to steer."
–George Bernard Shaw

Many physicians are hesitant when thinking about using advertising and selling techniques to promote their practice. If done correctly, these techniques can be very effective tools in establishing and enhancing a practice. To be effective, advertising must be:
- Directed at the target market.
- Advertising a service that the target market needs and wants.
- Professionally done.
- Sending the proper message.
- Given enough time to produce results.

Advertising and Selling

Advertising and selling are the on-going, long-term promotion of your practice. Advertising does have limits. Advertising cannot overcome unsatisfactory performance or create a demand when there is no need or want for the service.

Build the practice that you want by first defining what you want and then take the proper steps to obtain it. So far you have:
- Defined the practice that you want in your mission statement when you answered the question, "What is the purpose of my practice?"
- Defined your target markets when you answered the question, "Whom do you want as your customers?"
- Defined your competitive environment, when you answered the question, "Who are your competitors?"
- Defined your strengths, weaknesses, opportunities, and threats.
- Defined the goals of your practice, when you answered the question, "What do you want to accomplish in the practice?"
- Defined the needs and wants of the target market.
- Defined your service.
- Defined your fee schedule.

These are the foundations of your practice. Now, you need to communicate to your target markets who you are, what you do, and how you satisfy their needs and wants so they are motivated to become your customers.

In marketing, the communication of who you are, what you do, and how you satisfy the needs and wants of your target market is called the "message." The group of people that you contact in your target market is referred to as the "reach." Or, in other words, "Who do you reach when you run this ad?" How often that you reach your target market is referred to as "frequency." *Marketing is about reach and frequency to your target markets: who you reach and how often they hear your message.*

As a general rule, it takes at least three exposures to a message before anyone will act on that message. The more often the message is heard the more likely that the message will be

The Keys to Successful Marketing

acted upon. The initial announcement of a product or service is referred to as the "launch." When you launch a service you should have a high level of frequency. Once the product or service is launched, the frequency can be decreased.

In the first three months of practice, it is important to have at least three exposures to your target markets. Then use at least four more exposures to your target market in the next nine months of the first year. After the first year, the frequency can be decreased to three to four times a year. However, if you want to stimulate your practice to grow faster, increase the frequency and reach of your ads.

The following chapters discuss the mechanisms that you can use to reach your target markets including, marketing tools and ideas, and the use of media and public relations.

CHAPTER 9
Timing and Packaging

> *"Axiom 1: Timing is almost everything . . .
> Axiom 2: Packing is everything that timing is not."*
> –Robert Slaton, Ed.D., Bob Manning,
> and Clyde Jackson

> *"Nothing in this world is so powerful
> as an idea whose time has come."*
> –Victor Hugo

> *"Emerson said that if you build a better mousetrap the world will beat a path to your door, and that may have been true then . . . but it's not true now. No one will come. You have to package and promote that mousetrap. Then they will come."*
> –Charles Gillette

Timing and packaging are critical to your success. Successful practices interpret daily events, summarizing them into trends that are used to anticipate future events and seize opportunities. Knowing when to act is key to your success. Acting too early can force an idea before its time. Acting too late can miss an opportunity. If you are planning a marketing promotion, think about what else is going on in your community and time your advertising in accordance.

The Keys to Successful Marketing

Timing can also be used to stage a marketing campaign. For example, let's say you are sending a direct mail piece to all 2700 physicians in your community and your practice has two physicians and five office personnel. If you mail all 2700 pieces and receive a five percent response, you will receive 135 telephone calls. It will be very difficult to effectively handle this volume, thus creating a bad experience for your practice and the respondents. Instead of mailing all 2700 pieces at once, mail them in three of four batches spaced a week apart, thus spacing the 135 telephone calls over several weeks. Some examples of things that effect timing are:

- Vacation periods (July and August).
- National or Religious holidays (especially Christmas, Hanukah, Easter, Yom Kipper, and Thanksgiving).
- Major local events (e.g. sporting events, graduations, or festivals).
- What the competition is doing.
- Other events (e.g. the hospitals' medical staff holiday party or monthly staff meetings).

Marketing pieces that are professional, innovative, and properly packaged create interest and desirability. For example, if you are having a summer referring doctor party, wrap a professionally printed invitation around an ice cream cone and stuff the cone with large colored cotton balls that look like scoops of ice cream. Place this in a box and mail it as the invitation. Then at the event serve ice cream. Innovative packaging gets the recipient's attention and creates interest; people want to come to the party because they perceive that the party will be fun.

Use packaging to create a spin. For example, if you know a competitor is going to open a new pain center, pre-empt their announcement by sending a direct mail piece emphasizing your practice's proven track record and experience in successfully handing pain disorders.Use interesting packaging such as a picture of a running track or horse racing track and a tag line like, "While other are just getting into the race, we have been winning for over five years".

Timing and Packaging

Packaging can also overcome missed timing, but plain packaging is better than a marketing mistake. For example, sending an announcement card that is wrapped around a toy shovel containing the message, "We're breaking new ground in pain management," could convey the wrong message. The recipient may ask, "What are they shoveling?"

Sometimes both timing and packaging can go wrong. During the week of the 1996 Atlanta Olympic Games bombing, a hospital had sent a cardboard tube containing fake dynamite to local residents with the message, "We are exploding to serve you better." The hospital was demolishing a small building to create a new facility. Many residents who received the package telephoned the police. Luckily, the hospital pulled the campaign before all of the packages were sent. Needless to say, the campaign created negative publicity for the hospital.

The Keys to Successful Marketing

CHAPTER 10
Marketing Tools

"In the main, our competitors are acquainted with the same fundamental concepts and techniques and approaches that we follow, and they are free to pursue them as we are. More often than not, the difference between their level of success and ours lie in the relative thoroughness and self discipline with which we and they develop and execute our strategies for the future."
–Dick Neuschel

"The art of life lies in a constant readjustment to our surroundings"
–Kakuzo Okahura

There are several commonly used marketing tools: they are: announcement cards, business cards, appointment cards, reminder postcards, Rolodex® cards, brochures, introduction letters, educational packages, and newsletters. All marketing tools should contain your logo and use consistent colors and paper stock so that a consistent image is established which will enhance goodwill. However, it is acceptable to use different paper stocks based upon the use of the marketing tool. For example, your business cards, letterhead, and envelopes may be printed on white linen paper while your brochure is printed on glossy white paper.

Marketing Tools

Announcement

> "I don't know who you are.
> I don't know your company.
> I don't know your company's products.
> I don't know what your company stands for.
> I don't know your company's customers.
> I don't know your company's record.
> I don't know your company's reputation.
> Now — what was it you wanted to sell me?"
> –McGraw-Hill Publications

An announcement is sent to the medical community to inform them that you are now seeing patients and would like referrals to your practice. The announcement can also be made public by running ads in local newspapers, and on radio and/or television stations. When you run a public announcement, your costs escalate. *(For information on advertising in local newspaper, radio and/or television stations, see Media on pages 120-127.)*

Regardless of whether you decide to use public media or not, you should send out an announcement card to the entire medical community in your area, even if they are not in your target market. For example, if you are starting an acute, chronic, and cancer pain management practice, you will send an announcement card to physicians in your target market, such as orthopedic surgery, oncology, neurosurgery, neurology, occupational medicine, physical medicine and rehabilitation, internal medicine, rheumatology, and family practice. The announcement should also be sent to physicians who are not in your target markets, such as cardiology, general surgery, pathology, pulmonology, plastic surgery, gastroenterology, gynecology, hematology, otolaryngology, pediatrics, psychiatry, emergency medicine, and ophthalmology.

The names of people to whom you will send an announcement card should be compiled onto a mailing list. This mailing list can also used in the future for direct mailings (see pages 101-103).

The message on the announcement is the first exposure that the target market will have to your image. It is important that the message is professionally produced. Involve a graphic artist

The Keys to Successful Marketing

and/or professional marketing writers to assist in developing the message. The announcement card should communicate:
- Who you are.
- What you do.
- Where you practice.
- Other services that you offer that meet the needs and wants of the target market.

Announcement

The graphic artist can assist you in developing a professional graphic design for the announcement. The following pages show an example of an announcement.

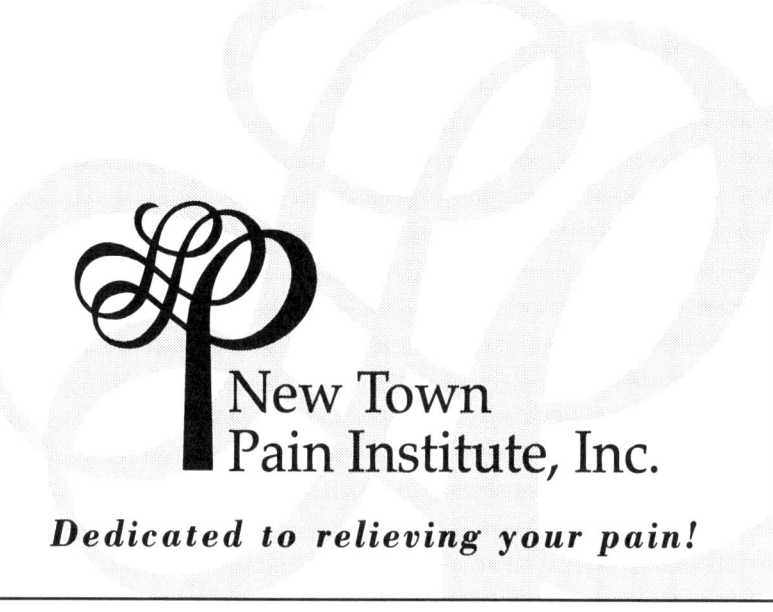

New Town Pain Institute, Inc.

Dedicated to relieving your pain!

Announcement Card — Front Cover

Marketing Tools

Drs Jones and Smith are proud to announce the formation of

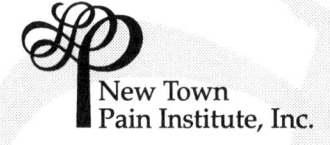

New Town
Pain Institute, Inc.

Dr. David C. Jones is board certified in both Anesthesiology and Pain Management by the American Board of Anesthesiology. He received his medical degree from Mount Sinai School of Medicine. He did his residency in Anesthesiology at Ohio State University and did his fellowship in Pain management at the Cleveland Clinic where he served as Chief Pain Fellow. His special interests include back pain and headache management.

Dr. Mary M. Smith is board certified in both Anesthesiology and Pain Management by the American Board of Anesthesiology. She received her medical degree from University of Chicago School of Medicine. She did her residency in Anesthesiology and fellowship in Pain management at the Cleveland Clinic. Her special interests include back pain and cancer pain management.

For more information about the New Town Pain Institute, or to schedule a patient to be seen and treated by a fellowship trained and board certified pain management expert, call:

(502) 555-1000

Springs Medical Plaza, 1000 Fifth Avenue, Suite 120, New Town, Kentucky 47772-4302

Announcement Card — Inside

Do not send the announcement until your clinical and business office is established. The last thing you want to have happen is to receive a referral from a physician for the first time and not be able to handle the referral or the patient professionally.

The Keys to Successful Marketing

Business Card

A business card is a professional way to give information to business or personal acquaintances. A business card should contain your name, logo, the name of your practice, and the address and phone number of your practice. In addition, you may also want to include your fax number and/or Internet address. An example of a business card is as follows:

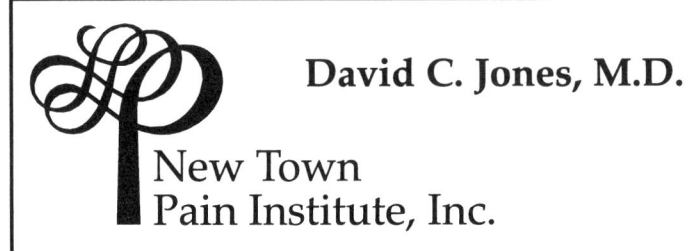

David C. Jones, M.D.

New Town
Pain Institute, Inc.

Springs Medical Plaza
1000 Fifth Avenue, Suite 120
New Town, Kentucky 47772-4302
Fax: (502) 555-1234
Phone: (502) 555-1000

Business Card

Appointment Cards

An appointment card is usually the size of a standard business card and is printed on both sizes. On one side is written the physician, practice name, address, and telephone number. The opposite side contains the date, time, and location that the patient will be seeing at the next appointment. This card is given out at the front desk when the patient leaves your office or by the referring doctor's office when they schedule a referral to your office. An example of an appointment card is as follows:

Marketing Tools

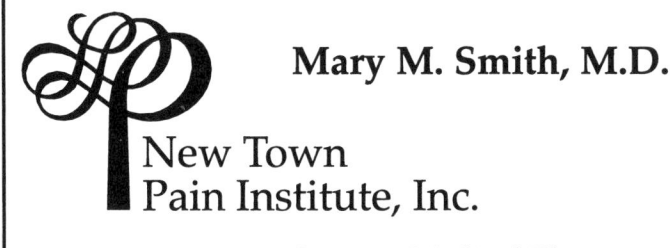

> **Mary M. Smith, M.D.**
>
> New Town
> Pain Institute, Inc.
>
> Springs Medical Plaza
> 1000 Fifth Avenue, Suite 120
> New Town, Kentucky 47772-4302
> Fax: (502) 555-1234
> Phone: (502) 555-1000

Appointment Card — Front Side

> **New Town Pain Institute Appointment**
>
> Date: _____
> Time: _____
>
> ❑ Springs Medical Plaza, 1000 Fifth Avenue, Suite 120
> ❑ Acme Regional Medical Center, 111 South Avenue
> ❑ New Town Hospital, One New Town Hospital Drive
> ❑ Lane Surgery Center, 6504 Oak Lane
>
> ***Dedicated to relieving your pain!***

Appointment Card — Reverse Side

Reminder Postcards

A reminder postcard is sent to patients to remind them of appointments that were scheduled several weeks or months in advance. For example, if a patient were scheduled to return in

The Keys to Successful Marketing

six months, then two to three weeks before the scheduled appointment a reminder postcard would be sent.

The reminder postcard lists the patient's appointment date, time, location, and the physician that they are scheduled to see as well as your practice's name, address, and phone number. Involve a graphic artist in designing the reminder postcard which should incorporate your logo, color choices, and positioning statement. The reminder postcard can be either automatically created by your scheduling computer software or hand-written. If the card is to be hand-written, create a postcard with blanks that can be filled in where appropriate. An example of a computer generated reminder postcard is as follows:

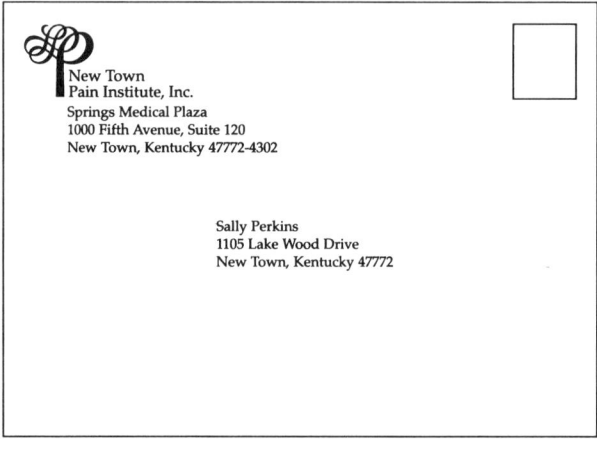

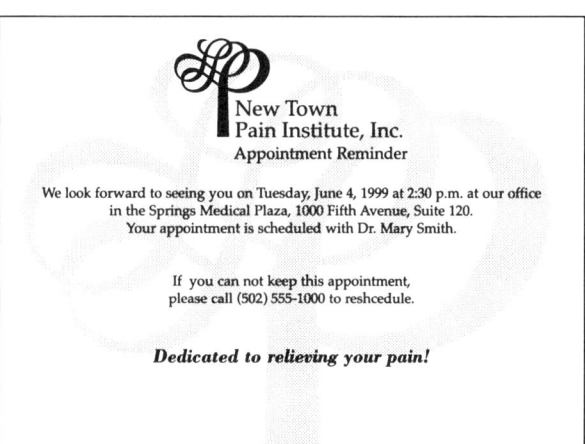

New Town
Pain Institute, Inc.
Springs Medical Plaza
1000 Fifth Avenue, Suite 120
New Town, Kentucky 47772-4302

Sally Perkins
1105 Lake Wood Drive
New Town, Kentucky 47772

New Town
Pain Institute, Inc.
Appointment Reminder

We look forward to seeing you on Tuesday, June 4, 1999 at 2:30 p.m. at our office in the Springs Medical Plaza, 1000 Fifth Avenue, Suite 120.
Your appointment is scheduled with Dr. Mary Smith.

If you can not keep this appointment,
please call (502) 555-1000 to reshcedule.

Dedicated to relieving your pain!

Computer Generated Reminder Post Card — Front and Reverse

Marketing Tools

An example of the contents of a form for a hand written reminder postcard is as follows:

```
New Town
Pain Institute, Inc.
Springs Medical Plaza
1000 Fifth Avenue, Suite 120
New Town, Kentucky 47772-4302
```

```
New Town
Pain Institute, Inc.

New Town Pain Institute
Appointment Reminder

We look forward to seeing you on: _____
                             At: _____
Your appointment is scheduled with: ❑ David C. Jones, M.D.  ❑ Mary M. Smith, M.D.

If you can not keep this appointment,
please call (502) 555-1000 to reschedule.

Dedicated to relieving your pain!
```

Hand Written Reminder Post Card — Front and Reverse

The Keys to Successful Marketing

Rolodex® Cards

Rolodex® cards are still widely used by most physician offices and managed care companies. The Rolodex® address filing system is stored in a variety of container systems with rings. Individual cards contain names, addresses, and phone numbers filed in alphabetical order. Rolodex® cards should be given to members of your target markets so that they can find you when they need you. An example of a Rolodex® card is as follows:

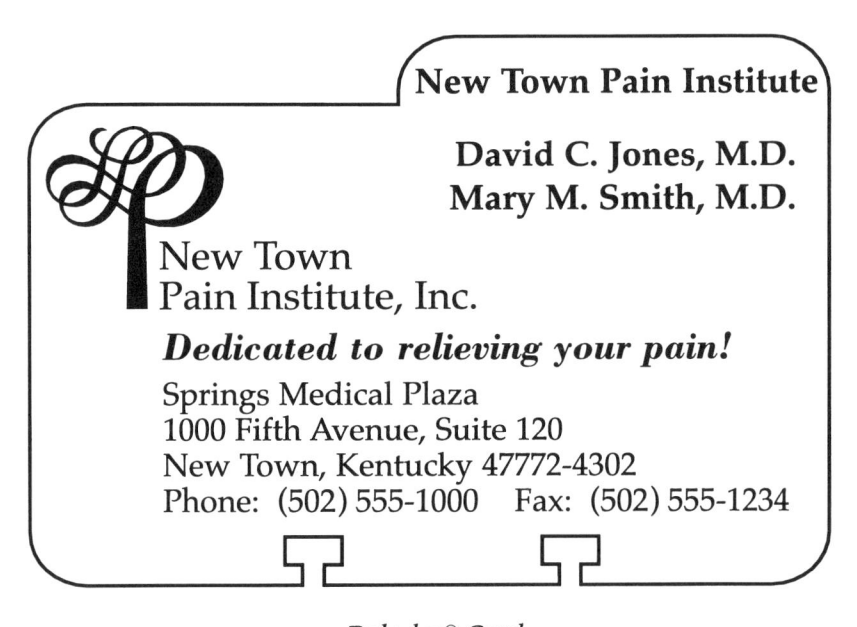

New Town Pain Institute

David C. Jones, M.D.
Mary M. Smith, M.D.

New Town
Pain Institute, Inc.

Dedicated to relieving your pain!

Springs Medical Plaza
1000 Fifth Avenue, Suite 120
New Town, Kentucky 47772-4302
Phone: (502) 555-1000 Fax: (502) 555-1234

Rolodex© Card

Brochures

A brochure is used to communicate to your target markets the following information:
- Who you are.
- What you do.
- Where you practice.

Marketing Tools

New Town
Pain Institute, Inc.

Dedicated to relieving your pain!

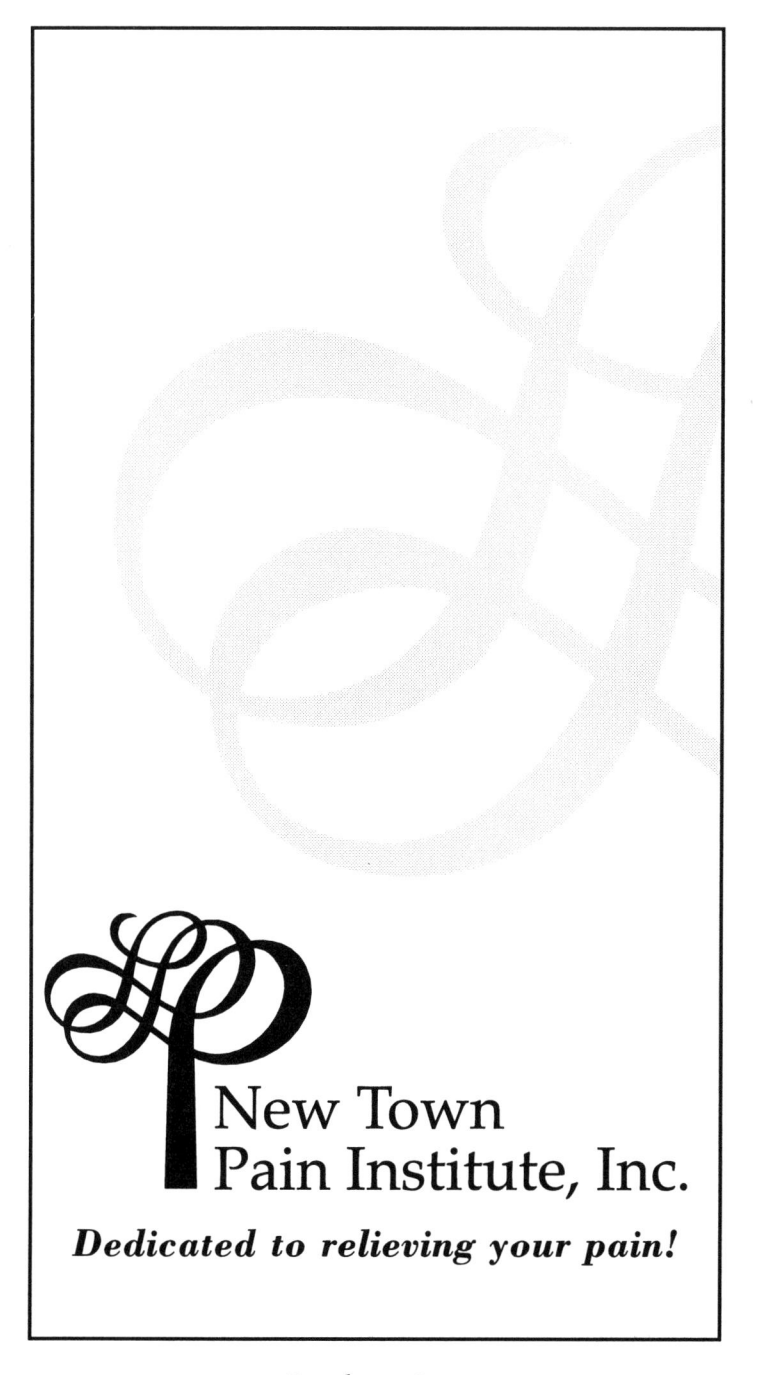

Brochure Cover

The Keys to Successful Marketing

The New Town Pain Institute is dedicated to relieving your pain!

Our physicians are board certified in both anesthesia and pain management. Pain management is a new board certifiable sub-specialty of anesthesia. It's a new approach to an age-old problem. At The New Town Pain Institute, we dedicate our entire practice to the prevention, evaluation, diagnosis, treatment, and rehabilitation of acute, chronic, and cancer pain disorders.

Pain disorders that we treat include:

- Back Pain
- Headache
- Cancer Pain
- Head and Neck Pain
- Neuralgia (including Shingles)
- Complex Regional Pain Syndrome (formerly called RSD)
- Causalgia
- Arthritis
- Facial Pain
- Post-Trauma Pain
- Rib Fracture Pain
- Musculoskeletal Pain

At The New Town Pain Institute we use a multidiscipline approach to treating your pain disorder. This approach can include one or more of the following:

- **Pain Relieving Procedures** including regional anesthesia injections and blocks, implantable and other devices including continuous epidural infusion, dorsal column stimulation, TENS units, spinal cord stimulation, and implantable infusion pump therapy
- **Medication Management**
- **Rehabilitation Services** including disability evaluations, physical therapy, occupation therapy, and acupuncture
- **Family and Patient Counseling** including education on pain disorders, biofeedback, relaxation training, and behavior modification

We are proud to provide inpatient and outpatient services at the following facilities:

- **Acme Regional Medical Center**
- **New Town Hospital**
- **Lane Surgery Center**

At The New Town Pain Institute we strive to relieve your pain so that you can return to the things you enjoy... traveling, reading, shopping, playing golf, cooking, gardening, playing tennis, exercising, working, in short normal daily activities that your pain disorder prevented you from doing. For more information about the New Town Pain Institute, or to schedule a patient to be seen and treated by a board certified pain management expert, call:

(502) 555-1000

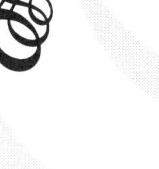

New Town Pain Institute, Inc.

New Town Pain Institute
Springs Medical Plaza,
1000 Fifth Avenue, Suite 120,
New Town, Kentucky 47772-4302

Inside Panels of Brochure

Marketing Tools

- Other services that you offer that meet the needs and wants of the target market.

The brochure is given to referring doctors' offices, patients, and managed care companies. Some referring doctors may also agree to keep a stack of your brochures in their reception area. An example of a brochure is on pages 95-96:

Introduction Letters

An introduction letter, much like the brochure, is sent to your target markets to communicate the following information:
- Who you are.
- What you do.
- Where you practice.
- Services that you offer that meets the needs and wants of the target market.

A marketing person or office manager will sign the letter. In addition to the introduction letter, you may also want to enclose a brochure, business card, and/or Rolodex® card in the mailing. An example of an introduction letter that might be sent to potential referring doctors is on the following page.

Educational Packages

An educational package is used to communicate information about pain management to a target market. The information is stored in a professionally printed folder your practice name, logo design, address, and telephone number. Inside the folder enclose articles which either you have written or which pertain to an area of interest to the target market. The articles should be professionally reprinted with permission from the publisher on glossy or other professional looking paper. If possible, avoid photocopies unless they are extremely professional looking. The

The Keys to Successful Marketing

New Town Pain Institute, Inc.

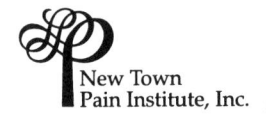

Dedicated to relieving your pain!

July 6, 1999

Dr. Ben White
5440 Long Lane
New Town, Kentucky 47777

Dear Dr. White;

Recently, there has been a lot of publicity and interest in the field of pain management. We at The New Town Pain Institute are proud to be the first medical practice in New Town that specializes exclusively in pain management, a new board certified specialty of anesthesia.

The New Town Pain Institute is comprised of a group of fellowship trained board certified Pain Management Anesthesiologists. We dedicate ourselves to relieving your patient's pain disorders. The physicians at The New Town Pain Institute are David Jones, M.D. and Mary Smith, M.D. Both physicians are fellowship trained and board certified in Anesthesiology and Pain Management by the American Board of Anesthesiology.

Dr. David Jones received his medical degree from Mount Sinai School of Medicine. He did his residency in Anesthesiology at Ohio State University and completed his fellowship in Pain Management at the Cleveland Clinic where he served as Chief Pain Fellow. His special interests include back pain and headache management.

Dr. Mary Smith received her medical degree from University of New Town School of Medicine. She did her residency in Anesthesiology and fellowship in Pain Management at the Cleveland Clinic. Her special interests include back pain and cancer pain management.

Enclosed is a brochure that explains our philosophy, the pain disorders that we treat, the services that we offer and the locations where we practice. For more information about the New Town Pain Institute, or to schedule a patient to be seen and treated by a fellowship trained and board certified pain management expert, call (502) 555-1000.

Sincerely,

Barbara Tucker
Director of Marketing

Springs Medical Plaza • 1000 Fifth Avenue, Suite 120 • New Town, Kentucky 47772-4302
Phone: (502) 555-1234 • Fax: (502) 555-1000

Introduction Letter

Marketing Tools

articles should emphasize pain management procedures that you perform and their success. Enclose a letter similar to the introductory letter but written to the target audience, along with a brochure, Rolodex® card, and business cards. An educational package is particularly helpful in markets where pain management is a new field and/or where your target markets may not be aware of the benefits of pain management treatment.

For example, if you are targeting oncologists, create an educational package that emphasizes the treatment options that you perform to successfully treat cancer pain. The purpose of this package is to communicate to the potential referring oncologist:

- You are knowledgeable in pain management.
- The definition and role of pain management as it applies to cancer pain management.
- Treatment options that they may not be aware of which can greatly relieve their patient's pain complaints.

Another example is an educational package targeted towards a managed care company. The folder should include articles containing general information on pain management treatment for many different pain disorders and, more importantly, articles that emphasize the cost-effectiveness of pain management treatment. You can also include the AHCPR (Agency for Healthcare Policy and Research) guidelines for the treatment of various pain disorders. Enclose a letter similar to the introductory letter but written to the managed care company, along with a brochure, Rolodex® card, and business cards. The purpose of this package is to communicate to the managed care company:

- You are knowledgeable in pain management.
- The general definition of pain management and its role in the successful treatment of various pain disorders.
- Pain management is a cost-effective treatment modality.

The Keys to Successful Marketing

Newsletters

A newsletter is an excellent mechanism to increase the frequency of exposures to your target markets and enhance your image and awareness in the community. As with all your published materials, the newsletter should contain your logo, practice name, address, and telephone number and be printed in your practice's color choices on good paper stock. Create a name and format for your newsletter. See page 103 for information on using bulk mail to get the most cost effective postage charges available.

As a guide, the newsletter should be approximately four pages in length and be published quarterly. Monthly publication should only be done if you have sufficient resources and informative articles. Even a quarterly newsletter requires a significant time commitment to produce. Before you commit to publishing a newsletter, you should make sure that you have sufficient qualified staff who can produce a professional newsletter. If you do not have the staff, you can hire external resources.

The newsletter should contain information that is interesting and informative to the reader. When you are deciding the content of the newsletter, consider who will be reading it. Will you be mailing the newsletter to patients, referring doctors, managed care companies, local employers, senior centers, hospital administrators, or all of these groups? Your target market will determine the content of the newsletter. You can write the articles, hire someone to write articles, or reprint articles from other published sources with the permission of the publisher. There are also companies that publish generic newsletters in all medical specialties and who will put your name and logo on a prepared newsletter.

The topics that you choose can vary widely. Generally the content of the newsletter should focus on the services that you want to provide. Some popular topics include patient testimonials, medical advances in diagnosing and treating a specific pain disorder, preventative health care, existing and new services, common pain complaints, and tips on avoiding reoccurrence of pain.

CHAPTER 11
Marketing Ideas

"Nothing levels a playing field like a better idea."
–Stanley I. Mason, Jr.

"Anything that you do to enhance sales is a promotion."
–Bill Veeck

All the marketing ideas discussed in this section have been successfully implemented by pain practices to help establish and grow their practices and increase goodwill.

Direct Mail

"If you want a thing done, go — if not, send."
–Benjamin Franklin

Direct mail is an effective method to reach your target markets. To start, choose one or more sources that sell computerized lists of your target markets. Mailing lists on diskette, mailing labels, or lists can be purchased or obtained from the following sources: county medical societies, hospitals, state boards of medical licensure, and state medical associations. In addition, you can rent mailing lists from direct mail companies. Some of

The Keys to Successful Marketing

these organizations will perform the mailing for a fee, but if possible, obtain the mailing lists on a diskette. If this is not possible, then obtain the list on mailing labels sorted by zip code and bar coded.

By using one or more of these sources, obtain a list of the physicians who are in your community and store it in a database. Then add to the database, referring physicians, hospital administrators, managed care company provider representatives, workers compensation caseworkers, personal friends, family members, and any other members of the target markets. Be sure to include in the database a relationship code, such as friend, physician, family member, etc.

The more people who are in the target markets that are on your mailing list, the greater the reach of your mailing. Depending on the mailing, you may want to include members of the medical community who are not in your target market. Since you are using a database, you can select the entire mailing list or just a sub-set such as family practice or internal medicine.

Most mailings should be sent only to your target markets, but mailings such as your announcement card should be send to the entire database. When you send out a mailing, keep track of what you sent and when you sent it.

Try to keep the database as current as possible. If you receive a change of address or address correction, change the address in the database. Annually, you should update your database with the national change of address. The national change of address can be purchased from one of several vendors who have contracted with the U.S. Post Office to record every change of address card that has been submitted to any U.S. Post Office.

The mailing list should contain the following information:
- Name, salutation (e.g. Dr., Mr., and Ms.) and suffix (e.g. M.D., Ph.D., R.N.). Having both the salutation and suffix allow more flexibility. For example, when mailing a letter address it to "Dr. Robert Smith" and when sending a post card address it to "Robert Smith, M.D."
- Street address (two lines), city, state, and zip code
- Telephone and fax numbers

Marketing Ideas

- Relationship type (e.g. physician, nurse, hospital administrator, friend, etc.)
- Specialty (e.g. orthopedics, family practice, internal medicine, etc.)
- Whether or not they have ever referred a patient; if yes, then the gross charges and net revenue referred.

When sending a direct mail piece, you must get the reader's attention immediately. Most practices receive dozens of direct mail promotions every day. The majority of them are thrown away before they are read. The chance of your brochure, newsletter, introduction letter, educational package, or other promotional piece being read is increased because it is a physician to physician correspondence. Your correspondence should make sure that this is readily apparent. Hire a professional advertising agency to develop eye catching and innovative material.

When sending out direct mail, have a bulk mail permit preprinted on the direct mail piece and use bar-coded addresses to get the cheapest postage available. While bulk mail is cheap, it can take a few days or even weeks to reach its destinations. The factors that effect the speed at which the mail arrives are the time of year, time of month, volume of mail, and distance that the mail will be traveling. The busiest mail period is during the holiday season. To find out more about timing bulk mail in your area, and to obtain a bulk mail permit, contact the U.S. Post Office branch near you. In order to use a bulk mail permit, the mail must be sorted in zip code order and bundled. Most practices use a mailing service to send out direct mail pieces to ensure that they conform to the postal rules and regulations.

Directories

"Never rest your oars. If you do, the whole company starts sinking."
–Lee Iacocca

Your target markets need to be able to find you. Patients may receive your number from a referring physician or from seeing

The Keys to Successful Marketing

or hearing advertisements that you have run. The most common way that a patient will find your telephone number is through the telephone book.

Referring physicians may find your telephone number from many different sources, including the telephone book, marketing literature, an advertisement, or a professional directory. It is important that you make it easy for them to find you.

Some directories are more expensive than others and some are free. As a general rule, the most expensive directory in which to purchase a listing is the Yellow Pages; however, it is the most likely place that someone will look for your phone number. At a minimum, you should have a bold listing in the Yellow Pages and a non-bold listing in the White Pages. A non-bold listing in the White Pages is free; you may want to consider purchasing a bold listing.

In some communities there is more than one company that publishes the Yellow Pages. Yellow Page publishers give telephone books away free, so some households and businesses will receive Yellow Pages from multiple sources. In order to determine in which books to be listed, find out which have the most usage. The Yellow Page publisher can tell you its demographics, but it is also helpful to think about the directories that you use, and ask others in the community which books they use. Purchase a listing in all of the books that are frequently used in your community.

Yellow and white page books are published annually. If you miss the cut-off for this year's books, you will have to wait an entire year before your practice can be listed in the directories. As soon as you start planning for your practice, find out when the cut-offs are and reserve a space.

Professional directories can also be a good source for referring physicians to find you. Depending on your community size, there can be a few or a dozen different directories. Some directories will publish your telephone number and address for free; others will charge you to be listed. As a general rule, you can be listed in a directory for free if you are a member of that group. Consider running ads in directories where your target markets

Marketing Ideas

are members. Most directories are published annually; if possible, get into this year's directory. Some important directories to be listed in are:
- Medical rosters at the hospitals where you are on staff.
- Insurance companies with whom you participate.
- County medical societies to which you belong.
- State medical societies to which you belong.
- Professional associations to which you belong such as American Society of Anesthesiologists, American Medical Association, American Academy of Pain Medicine, Society of Pain Practice Management, American Pain Society, and the American Society of Regional Anesthesia.
- Professional associations to which you do not belong, but your target markets do belong, such as the your state's chapter of the Association of Family Physicians, the Association of Internal Medicine, the Registered Nurses Association, etc.

Listing in the directories in which your target markets are a member increases the potential frequency that a member will see and remember your practice. If they remember you, goodwill is increased and they could refer a patient.

Promotional Items

"We despise no source that can pay us a pleasing attention."
–Mark Twain

Promotional items are any items imprinted with your logo and position statement that you give away to promote your practice. There are thousands of promotional items available. In addition to canvas bags, coffee cups and pens, some of the more common promotional items include:
- Hats
- Shirts
- Drink Holders

The Keys to Successful Marketing

- Frisbees
- Magnets
- Post-it Notes

You can, for a price, have your logo and positioning statement imprinted on just about anything you can think of. When you are evaluating promotional items to purchase, you need to consider three things:
- Initial impact on your target market.
- Continued impact on your target market.
- Cost.

The most important factor is the impact your item will have on your target market. What will they think when they receive this item? Will they use the item or discard it? Will they continue to use it day after day? Will the use of the item enhance goodwill and stimulate your business? Remember that you want the target market to see your image frequently so your practice and services are always in their minds. The image that they see should be favorable.

There are two items that are low cost and very effective – the coffee cup and the pen. The coffee cup is low cost, less than $1.50 each for a white cup printed with two colors on two sides. A coffee cup has a high impact because it looks more expensive than it is. If used, the person using it is drinking coffee or tea out of it everyday. The pen is also low cost, around $.50 each for a standard white Bic Click® pen printed with one color of ink. The pen also has a high continued impact because the person using it is writing with it everyday. Unfortunately, the pen will eventually run out of ink, and unlike the coffee cup, it will be thrown away. Therefore, the coffee cup has a higher and longer-term impact than the pen. Both the coffee cup and pen are items that are commonly given away because of their marketing strengths.

Depending upon your community, you may want to choose an item that may be less cost-effective but has a higher initial impact, for example a hat, t-shirt, or polo shirt that has been

Marketing Ideas

imprinted with your logo and positioning statement. These items look expensive because on the relative scale, they are expensive — often these items cost more than $15.00 each. But they have high impact because people recognize that they were costly.

Professional Societies

> *"Accept the challenges, so that you may feel the exhilaration of victory."*
> –George Patton

Professional societies often have regular educational meetings that you can participate in by being a speaker and/or a vendor. Giving a lecture is a wonderful way to demonstrate your medical expertise and increase your exposure to members of the target markets who will remember your practice, thus increasing your goodwill.

There are also many ways to participate in the educational meetings of professional groups by being a vendor. You can have a booth; sponsor an event, such as a breakfast, lunch, cocktail party or dinner; or provide promotional items such as canvas bags, coffee cups, pens, or hats that are handed out to the meeting participants. Participating as a vendor is more expensive than being a speaker, but still offers one of the most cost-effective methods of having one-on-one conversations with members of your target markets. When talking with members of your target group, you should communicate the following message: who you are, what you do, where you practice, and what services you offer.

Professional societies pay for the majority of the cost of the meeting by having vendors. The cost of having a booth usually includes a piped and draped booth in a certain dimension (e.g. 8' x 10'), a draped table, and two chairs. Sometimes the booth will also include an electrical outlet and carpeting. Be sure to ask what is included in the booth because there will be a charge for additional items.

The Keys to Successful Marketing

Think about how your booth will look. There are companies that make professional display units that you can put in the booth. At a minimum, you need to have a professional sign that can be hung in the booth or placed on an easel. The sign should contain the following information: who you are, what you do, where you practice, and what services that you offer. As with all printed material, the sign should use your logo, color choices, and position statement.

Promotional items and educational literature in the booth helps to further communicate your message and image. Have plenty of brochures, newsletters, business cards, Rolodex® cards, promotional items, and educational packages to give to all attendees of the meeting. During the meeting, be sure that the staff manning the booth is knowledgeable, professional, and competent in effectively communicating who you are, what you do, where you practice, and what services that you offer.

Presentations to Target Markets

"No great thing is suddenly created.'"
–Epictetus

Another method of demonstrating your medical expertise is to give presentations to your target markets on topics that are informative and interesting to them. Speaking at professional societies such as the American Society of Anesthesiologists, American Academy of Pain Medicine, American Society of Regional Anesthesia, Society of Pain Practice Management, state or county medical associations, state nurses' associations, occupational rehabilitation nurses associations, and/or workers compensation caseworkers will promote both you and your practice. Volunteer to speak at medical staff meetings, workers compensation insurance company meetings, health education programs sponsored by the hospital, or support groups for patients who have cancer or chronic headaches.

Decide on a topic that you can easily speak about for an extended time. If you don't choose a topic, one will be chosen for

Marketing Ideas

you that you may not be comfortable speaking about. The topic can be anything that interests your target markets. For example, a lecture could be on "The Five Most Common Back Complaints and their Treatments," or, "You Don't Have to Live with Your Pain: An Introduction to Pain Management." Make the topic exciting so people will attend the lecture.

Have one to four polished speeches that you know well. Put together a presentation that contains your best possible educational materials and anecdotes so that it can be delivered in the shortest time possible, adding restrained humor to make it entertaining and memorable. Create a professional presentation using 35mm color slides or computer-generated color storyboards. Pay close attention to the choice of colors because some colors schemes are not easily seen from the back of the room. Also, incorporate on every slide your practice logo and color choices into the presentation. Create and distribute paper handouts of your slides. This increases the frequency that your practice has exposure to the target market, thus increasing goodwill.

In order to obtain speaking engagements identify groups in your target markets. Contact the organizations' leaders, ask when and where their next meeting is, and if they would like to have you lecture on the pain management topic that you have selected. Usually, they will ask you to send some professional history information or synopsis of your lecture. Promptly respond to this request. If the organizations' leaders find your topic interesting, they will invite you to be a speaker.

The chances of obtaining a speaking engagement are increased if your topic is interesting and you are willing to speak for free; however, some groups are very willing to pay you an honorarium to speak. In addition, organizations such as drug companies, home health agencies, hospitals, rehabilitation centers, and medical equipment suppliers may be willing to sponsor you. They are willing to pay for your time and travel expenses because they want to create a program that is beneficial to their target markets thus promoting their products and/or services. Sponsor organizations keep a list of recommended speakers and will offer you many paid speaking engagements throughout the

The Keys to Successful Marketing

country, and possibly internationally. As your reputation develops, you will find it easier and easier to obtain paid speaking engagements. You and your practice's fame will grow.

When giving a speech, know your audience. Confirm the number of participants and bring more handouts and marketing materials than there are participants. Often audience members will take an extra copy of your handouts or marketing materials back to another member of your target market. Determine audiovisual needs and make arrangements prior to your lecture. Prepare a brief summary of your qualifications including education, work experience, accomplishments, offices held, board certification, and present professional position that can be read by the person who is introducing you. When you speak, be sure that your appearance is professional. Wear a traditionally-styled dark colored business suit, and if male, a collared shirt and tie, even if your audience is dressed casually. Arrive early and verify that the audiovisual equipment and microphones are present and operational and then coach the person who will be introducing you on your background.

During the lecture, maintain eye contact with the audience, assess their involvement, and adjust your lecture accordingly. Use questions to involve the audience and make sure the meeting environment is comfortable. The room temperature should be pleasant, give stretch and restroom breaks as needed, and ask for refreshments to be provided. Repeat participants' questions before answering them so that other members of the audience hear the question being answered. Keep on schedule, arrive early, start and end on time, and stay late to answer audience questions. At the conclusion of the lecture, cue the person who introduced you to close the lecture.

New Physicians

"Companies don't make purchases; they establish relationships."
–Charles S. Goodman

Marketing Ideas

It is important that when a new physician who is a member of your target market begins practicing in your community that you make her/him aware of your practice and the services that it offers. There are several ways to find out who the new doctors are in your community. New doctors usually send out an announcement card, or are mentioned in the hospitals' medical staff newsletter and/or county or state medical society newspapers and magazines.

Introduce yourself by sending a letter or an item for their office welcoming them to practice. For example, send a potted plant with fresh flowers and a note simply stating, "Wishing you success." The potted plant will usually be placed somewhere in their office and will provide a constant reminder of your hospitality. Within the first month that they are in practice, send an introduction letter, brochure and/or educational package explaining your services to them, or make an office visit. See pages 112-114 for information on *Marketing Office Visits*.

In addition, you can introduce yourself by taking the new physician to lunch. This gives you an extended period of time to not only conduct business, but to establish a professional friendship. Chances are that when a new doctor is starting in practice, her/his patient schedule is light and she/he has a lot of time available to go to lunch. If you take a new physician to lunch you need to:

- Be on time. Be considerate of the new physician's time and conclude the lunch on time.
- Try not to cancel the lunch. If a medical emergency prevents you from attending the lunch at the last minute, call and send someone else from your practice who can "talk the talk and walk the walk."
- Go to a quiet and good restaurant in a location that is convenient for the new physician.
- Ask about and listen to what the new physician is doing.
- Do not drink alcoholic beverages during business hours.
- Pay for the lunch.

Casual Conversations and The Doctors' Lounge

> *"Friendship founded on business is better than a business founded on friendship."*
> –John D. Rockefeller, Jr.
>
> *"A fellow doesn't last long on what he has done. He's got to keep on delivering as he goes along."*
> –Carl Hebbell

Physician-to-physician contact is the best way to explain who you are, what you do, and establish a professional relationship with physicians in your target markets. Make it a goal to attend every medical staff meeting and to meet potential referring physicians. Whenever you are not busy seeing and/or treating patients and you are at a hospital or surgery center that has a doctors' lounge, take time to stop in and chat with the physicians who are there. Talk about anything that is socially, morally, and ethically acceptable. Make a special point to meet new physicians and key members of your target market, such as the orthopedic surgeon who schedules a lot of surgeries, or the busy internal medicine physician who admits a lot of patients.

Developing professional relationships will help build your practice. Chances are if you take time to talk to a physician face to face, the physician will remember you and might refer to you. Remember, marketing is about reach and frequency: who you reach and how frequently that they hear your message.

Once a bond of camaraderie and a trust level is established, you will begin to receive referrals. Be sure to return the favor with your own referrals, see pages 115-119 for more information on outgoing referrals. Continue to meet their needs and their patients needs and you will establish a long-term professional relationship that will be difficult for competitors to undermine.

Marketing Office Visits

> *"Since not all tasks are created equal, the organized executive must set priorities: that is, establish a hierarchy of importance, and match the commitment of time and resources to the relative importance of each task".*
> –Stephanie Winston

Marketing Ideas

It is important that the physicians and their staff who are in your target markets know who you are and what you do. As discussed previously, one of the best ways to communicate to your target physicians is by physician-to-physician conversation. But this type of communication takes time, and it is not feasible for you to meet the entire medical community, including the potential referring physician's office staff.

One of the best ways to get exposure is to have an office manager or marketing person drop by the potential referring physician's offices with marketing literature about your practice, promotional items, and/or a treat (cookies, muffins, donuts, or candy). The marketing person or office manager must be knowledgeable in pain management and be able to effectively communicate the services that are offered by your practice. This method has been used by most prescription drug companies for many years and continues to be used because it is successful.

In order to make the best use of time, carefully select and prioritize the physicians in your target markets. Determine which specialties of physicians are most likely to refer the most patients. Then prioritize the individual physicians or medical groups within the specific specialties.

For example, let's assume that you believe that most of your referrals will come from orthopedic surgery. Obtain a list of all of the orthopedic surgeons and orthopedic surgery group practices in your community. Let's assume that there are 74 orthopedic surgeons in your community who practice in 26 groups of one or more physicians. Prioritize these 26 practices by the number of orthopedic surgeons in the group so that you will call on the groups with the highest number of orthopedic surgeons first. Then decide what type of office visit you are going to schedule. Is your representative going to stop by unannounced with donuts, candy, brownies, popcorn or some other treat? Or, will she/he call ahead, schedule a visit, and bring that staff lunch?

Since you believe that orthopedic surgeons will send the most referrals, you decide to have your representative take lunch to the physicians and their staff. Have your representative call the office manager, inform her/him that your practice is interested in bringing lunch for the physicians and their staff and ask if there is a date that would be convenient for them. Some groups may not wish to have lunch brought into them, while other groups will be pleased with this offer. Once you agree upon a date, ask if there are any dietary considerations that you need to know. Be sure to find your how many people will be having lunch and whether or not the office has a lunchroom and ice.

Have your representative call the chosen restaurant well in advance of the date, inquire if the restaurant will deliver, and make the appropriate arrangements. Then she/he should confirm the arrangements and headcount the day before the visit with the restaurant and the physician's office. When the date arrives, she/he should bring or have the food delivered and make sure there are enough beverages, cups, utensils (forks, spoons, plates, and napkins), and ice. In addition, she/he should bring marketing literature and promotional items including business cards, Rolodex® cards, brochures, educational packages, coffee cups, and/or pens.

During the lunch, your representative should be available to talk about the practice and answer questions. As a general rule, she/he should not eat during the luncheon and should conclude the lunch and leave after everyone has eaten. Remember that most offices have staggered lunch breaks, so that there is coverage on the telephones so the lunch period will usually span two hours.

Once your representative has finished this lunch, she/he should continue to conduct lunches until all 26 offices have been called upon. Generally, you can realistically schedule about three lunches per week, so expect this process to take about two months. Then you should determine your next target group, for example, internal medicine and family practice. Prioritize the practices and call on those offices perhaps taking bagels or muffins, which are considered healthier than donuts or pastries. This activity can be simultaneous to conducting lunches for orthopedic groups. Continue to call on offices until all groups in your target markets have been called upon. Repeat office calls for groups who either refer, or could refer, many patients.

Marketing Ideas

Outgoing Referrals

> *"Hitch your wagon to a star."*
> –Ralph Waldo Emerson

> *"Government is not the solution to our problem. Government is the problem."*
> –Ronald Reagan

Referring a patient to another physician is another way to get to know that physician. If, for example, you have a patient who is a candidate for orthopedic surgery, refer that patient to an orthopedic surgeon who either is, or could be, a potential referring doctor. Remember that the most important decision in making a referral is medical necessity and the competence of the physician to whom you are referring. Do not expect anything in return and do not make any referral arrangements that could violate The Federal Anti-Kickback Statute and the Ethics in Patient Referrals Act (commonly referred to as Stark Legislation).

THE FEDERAL ANTI-KICKBACK STATUTE

Enacted in 1972, and amended in 1977, 1987 and 1991, the "The Federal Anti-Kickback Statute" was created to help prevent "remuneration (including any kickbacks, bribes, or rebates)" for referrals in the Medicare or Medicaid program either "directly or indirectly, overtly or covertly, in cash or in kind." This statue prohibits any kind of economic incentives for referrals including barter and monetary arrangements. Each violation of this statute is a felony, punishable by a fine of up to $25,000 and imprisonment of up to five years. Even if no criminal conviction has been obtained, the Secretary of Health and Human Services may exclude violators from participation in Medicare and Medicaid. Civil monetary penalties are also at the disposal of the secretary.

In 1989, Congress mandated that the Office of Inspector General promulgate regulations to specify certain referral arrangements that are permissible under the law. Issued in 1991,

The Keys to Successful Marketing

these regulations detail the "safe harbors" of conduct that are exempt from The Federal Anti-Kickback Statute. The categories of conduct addressed by the safe harbors include:
- Investments in publicly-traded companies
- Investment in small businesses
- Personnel services/management agreements
- Sale of professional practices
- Referral services
- Warranties
- Discounts
- Employment
- Group purchasing
- Co-insurance
- Space rentals
- Equipment rentals

The Secretary of Health has issued several advisory opinions concerning the meaning of the statute and these regulations. Contact an attorney who specializes in The Federal Anti-Kickback Statute if you need advice on this law.

ETHICS IN PATIENT REFERRALS ACT
(STARK LEGISLATION)

Congressman Pete Stark, believing that The Federal Anti-Kickback Statute was incomplete, proposed legislation to restrict a physician from referring Medicare and Medicaid patients for designated health services to an entity in which the physician or an immediate family member of the physician has ownership. However, these restrictions do not apply to referrals for services furnished personally by a physician in the same group practice as the referring physician or for services furnished by another physician under the personal supervision of a physician in the same group practice as the referring physician. Congressman Stark's proposed restrictions were passed by congress and became effective in late 1994 via the Ethics In Patient Referrals Act. The Health Care Finance Administration (HFCA) has pub-

lished two sets of final regulations aimed at clarifying this Act, which is commonly referred to as the Stark Legislation. The definition of designated health services includes:
- Physical therapy services, such as traditional outpatient physical therapy aimed at the prevention of pain or disability. These services include a wide range of diagnostic procedures including tests that measure neuromuscular, musculoskeletal, cardiovascular, and pulmonary function. This definition applies to most comprehensive pain management programs and CORF (comprehensive outpatient rehabilitation facilities).
- Radiology services, including MRI, CAT scan, and ultrasound.
- Outpatient prescription drugs, including all prescription drugs and biologicals administrated under a physician's supervision that can be obtained by prescription from a pharmacy.
- Clinical laboratory services.
- Occupational therapy services.
- Radiation therapy services and supplies.
- Durable medical equipment and supplies.
- Parenteral and enteral nutrients, equipment, and supplies.
- Prosthetics, orthotics, and prosthetic devices and supplies.
- Home health services.
- Inpatient and outpatient hospital services.

As stated above, Stark's prohibition on referral does not apply to certain activities in group practice settings. A group practice is defined as a group of two or more physicians who are legally organized as a partnership, professional corporation, foundation, non-profit corporation, faculty practice, plan, or other similar association. Stark's regulations presume that a group can be composed of several single physicians who are individually incorporated as professional corporations. All group practices are subject to the following conditions:

The Keys to Successful Marketing

- Physicians must share office space, facilities, equipment, and personnel, and each physician in the group must provide a full range of services including medical care, consultation, diagnosis, and treatment that the referring physician provides.
- At least 75% of the total patient care services rendered by all the physician members of the group must be billed under a billing number assigned to that group. Groups must operate as a centralized and unified business.
- Physician compensation must be distributed in accordance with methods that are adopted prior to the period during which the income is earned or the expense is incurred. This payment method cannot compensate any member based upon the volume or value of that member's referrals. Productivity bonuses are allowed as long as there is no direct linkage to the volume or value of referrals.

In-office ancillary services also qualify as an exception to Stark's prohibition. Although parenteral and enteral nutrition and durable medical equipment are not protected within this exception, by statute's terms, referrals for infusion pumps and crutches can quality. To qualify for the in-office ancillary services exception these conditions must be met:

- The referring physician must be a member of the same group practice that provides and supervises the designated health service rather than an independent contractor.
- The designed health services must be furnished in the same building as the referring physician furnished services unrelated to the designated health service or in another building utilized by the group for centralized designed health services (the building must have the same address, not multiple structures connected by tunnels or walkways).
- The services must be billed:
    a. By the physician who performed or supervised the services.
    b. By the group practice that employs the physician.

Marketing Ideas

c. By a wholly owned entity of the group practice.

This Act also exempts salaried physicians who are employed by the group or hospital. Employment agreements between hospitals and physicians must meet the following requirements:
- The employment agreement must be in writing and be signed by both parties.
- Services to be rendered must be enumerated in the agreement.
- The physician's salary must be consistent with fair market value for the services in an arm's-length transaction and not based upon the volume or value of referrals.
- The physician's salary must be commercially reasonable even if no referrals were made to the hospital.

Contact an attorney who specializes in Stark Legislation if you need advice on these laws.

Seasonal or Occasional Correspondence

"There are no traffic jams when you go the extra mile."
–Anonymous

In marketing you are trying to get your message to your target markets as frequently as possible. Take advantage of any reasonable opportunity that you can seize upon to keep your message in your target markets' minds, such as sending a holiday card, birthday card, holiday gift, and/or having a referring doctor party.

The Keys to Successful Marketing

CHAPTER 12
Media

"Advertising is like learning — a little is a dangerous thing."
–P. T. Barnum

"If you have an important point to make, don't try to be subtle or clever. Use a pile driver. Hit the point once. Then come back and hit it again. Then hit it a third time — a tremendous whack."
–Winston Churchill

When most people think of advertising, they think about communicating their message via media. Media consists of print, sound, and a combination of sound and picture. These formats are available from many sources including newspapers, billboards, magazines, radio, television (both regular and cable), and the Internet. While some media may have very specific target markets, others are targeted towards the general public.

The medium you select will determine the style, content, and length of your ad. The ad can be educational, informative, or a testimonial. All of your advertisements should contain the following information:

- Who you are, where you are located, and how to get in contact with you (your practice name, logo, address, and telephone numbers).
- What services you offer and how they are beneficial to the target market.
- Why you are better than your competition.
- What days and hours that your office is open.
- A call to action (act now).

In any advertising medium, the most important aspect is that you communicate your message to your target markets frequently enough that they will remember you. Most people need at least three exposures to a message before they will remember it.

Some media, such as radio and television stations, conduct extensive research of their audience demographics. Others, such as the major newspaper in your community, reach a more public audience. In any case, find out as much as you can about the media's audience before you advertise with them.

It is also important that your message communicates what you want to say properly. Involve an advertising agency to assist you in developing a professional ad campaign that is consistent no matter what medium you employ. A professional and consistent message will increase the probability that your target markets will remember your message, thus increasing goodwill.

Advertising is the most expensive way to communicate your message, and you need frequency to accomplish results. If you do not have the financial resources for frequent advertising, then use other marketing techniques. It is a waste of your money to run infrequent ads.

In addition to the cost of running the ad, there is also a cost associated with developing an ad. Create a good campaign and then use it over again for several years with different providers in the same medium. Most media providers will assist you in creating the ad, but if they do, you will not be able to use the ad with other providers. Most media providers will give you a discount if you develop your own ad. The costs associated with running ads are negotiable, and discounts are based upon fre-

The Keys to Successful Marketing

quency and/or volume. If you are unable to negotiate a cash discount, ask for additional ad placements to be thrown in free of charge. To get the best discounts, plan and commit to an ad campaign that runs for an entire year.

Newspapers and Newsletters

> "Advertisements contain the only truths to be relied on in a newspaper."
> –Thomas Jefferson

Most communities have one main newspaper and several smaller newspapers and newsletters. The smaller newspapers and newsletters generally have a specific target group that is a sub-set of a larger community, such as:
- A particular religion, such as Catholic, Jewish, or Baptist.
- A smaller community or neighborhood.
- An age group, such as teenagers or senior citizens.
- Specific interests, such as doll collecting, antique collecting, fishing, sailing, or tennis.
- Diseases, such as cancer, headaches, diabetes, muscular dystrophy, or arthritis.

If one of these papers serves a market niche that you are interested in serving, run an ad. Printed ads when published in reputable newspapers often have a great deal of creditability because the people will believe what they read. Since the ad is hard copy, people often cut them out and refer back to them. In addition, a single copy of a newspaper or newsletter is often read by more than one person. Print advertising allows you to communicate a lot of information, but be careful not to lose the reader's interest by providing too much detail.

Newspaper and newsletter ads are priced based upon circulation, placement, and size of the ad. Generally, the higher the circulation, the more public placement (e.g. back page, front page of the health section), the larger the ad, the more expensive it will be. Placement within the newspaper can be an important decision because different people read certain sections. The main section of the newspaper is the most commonly read. A predominately female audience usually reads the lifestyle section, and the sports section is usually read by a predominately male audience. Never assume that because a newspaper has a high circulation that it will be read by your target market. It is more important to reach your target market than to reach the masses.

Billboards

"The guy you've really got to reach with your advertising is the copywriter for your chief rival's advertising agency. If you can terrorize him, you've got it licked."
–Howard L. Gossage

Billboards are outdoor signs that reach people who travel along the roads where they are located. In most cases a billboard is stationary, but in some cases the billboard is mobile, such as a billboard on the side of a bus or on a mobile trailer. The message on billboards should be in large print and very simple. Most people will only have a few seconds to read the billboard and understand the message. Billboards are priced based upon the location of the billboard and the size of the ad. Mobile billboards can be placed in a specific location such as a parking lot. In general, the more public the location, such as on a main expressway or major roadway, and the larger the board, the more expensive the ad.

Magazines

"Nothing but the mint can make money without advertising."
–Thomas B. Macaulay

Like newspapers, magazines contain printed advertisements that enhance creditability because people believe what they read.

The Keys to Successful Marketing

Magazines, also like newspapers, allow you to communicate a lot of information and are often read by more than one person. But unlike newspapers that are discarded within the first few days of publication, magazines are often kept for a long period of time, thus increasing the probability that your ad could be read again or by another person. Like newspaper ads, magazine ad costs are based upon circulation, placement, and size of the ad.

Radio

> "The codfish lays 10,000 eggs.
> The homely hen just one;
> The codfish never crackles
> To tell you that she's done.
> And so we scorn the codfish,
> And the homely hen we prize.
> Which demonstrates to you and me
> That it pays to advertise."
> –The Toronto Globe

Radio is listened to by a wide variety of people in many places. A radio station may be playing in a person's car, in an office, or at a shopping mall. Since a radio spot is heard and not seen, the listener will need more exposures to a message than with print advertising. The message in a radio ad should be quick and simple. If the listener did not understand the message, then she/he will move onto the next piece of music or news story.

Your radio ad can be prerecorded in a professional sound studio or read live by the announcer. If you decide to have a prerecorded ad, you need to consider whether you want a male or a female voice. In addition, you may have individuals in your community whose voices are readily recognized. Using a local celebrity such as a newscaster or health authority can provide instant creditability to your advertisement.

Radio spots are sold in 30- or 60-second increments. The spots are sold based upon the number of listeners who are listening during certain time periods and the length of the spot. As a general rule, you will pay more for advertising during time periods where there are more listeners tuned in, for example during the morning and evening drive times, and noon-hour news programs. The spots that are in the early morning hours, like 3:00 a.m., often are thrown in for little or no additional cost when you are purchasing other time spots. Radio stations also conduct extensive research into their audience demographics. Ask for an audience profile before committing to a contract.

Public radio stations offer an inexpensive method to reach a small but well-educated audience. Most cities have more than one public radio station and offer discounts if you advertise on every public radio station. Depending upon the station, the programming format maybe all news, classical music, jazz, or a combination of many programs. Public radio does not allow advertisement, but instead has sponsorships. The announcer will read a statement such as, "The news was brought to you by The New Town Pain Institute, dedicated to relieving your pain."

In addition to the cost of airing the radio spot, there may be costs associated with creating the spot. Involve a professional advertising agency and create a quality spot that can be used for several years on several different stations. Many radio stations will assist you in developing a spot, but if the radio station develops the spot, you will not be able to use it on other stations. Most radio stations will give you a discount if you develop your own ad.

Television (Regular and Cable)

"Some people make headlines while others make history."
–Phillip Elmer-DeWitt

Television is the most successful medium to reach the masses. The four network stations are ABC, CBS, NBC, and Fox, and there are many other cable TV stations that offer programs which target specific interest areas. For example, CNBC broadcasts business news, CNN is an all-news format,

The Keys to Successful Marketing

and Lifetime is devoted to programming for adult women. Pricing is based upon the number of viewers, the length of the spot, the time of day, and the station selected. As a general rule, cable TV stations charge less than the network stations. Television spots for programs that are very popular are the most costly.

If you are considering advertising on television, but have a limited budget, find out if there is a local cable TV station that has a medical or preventative healthcare related segment. This can be a cost-effective alternative in communicating your message. Like radio stations, television stations conduct extensive marketing research on who is watching their programming at given time periods throughout the day and night. Most stations can provide an audience profile in 30-minute increments. And like radio, TV spots in the early morning hours are very cost-effective. While this should not be your primary time slot for running a television ad, consider purchasing some of the early morning time spots because people who are in pain are often unable to sleep and might turn on the television in the early hours.

Most television spots are 15, 30, or 60 seconds in length. This short time period limits how much you can communicate, but remember that a picture can say a thousand words. Like radio, the impact of your message may be quickly forgotten. It is only with frequency and creativity that you will be able to achieve a message that the viewers will remember. In addition to the cost of airing the television spot, there may be significant costs associated with creating the spot. Involve a professional advertising agency and create a good spot that can be used for several years on several different stations. Like radio, television stations will develop a spot, but will not allow you to use it on other stations. Most television stations will give you a discount if you develop your own ad.

Internet

"Mighty things from small beginnings grow."
–John Dryden

Media

The Internet is the only advertising medium that allows you to have customized interactive two-way graphical and verbal communication with the individuals in your target market. The Internet allows you to create a web site where you can store information about your practice and the services that you offer. The information can be comprehensive but should be layered to allow the user the ability to conveniently select the information that is relevant to his or her needs. The user can also ask you direct questions via electronic mail, or using more sophisticated software, the user can telephone your practice from their computer on the internet.

Hire a professional to set up your web site and designate someone on your staff to keep the site operational, and to read and answer e-mail messages. Make sure that the person you hire links your site to plenty of other sites and search engines in order to get many visitors to your site.

CHAPTER 13
Public Relations

"Get someone else to blow your horn and the sound will carry twice as far."
–Will Rogers

Public relations is defined as the act of fostering pubic goodwill toward an individual or an entity. Public relations differs from advertising because you do not control the message and you do not pay for the public exposure. If the message is positive, public relations can provide more creditability than advertising because the message is coming from an independent third-party source. The reader, listener, or viewer of a news story will interpret the story to be authentic and without bias.

Public relations used in conjunction with advertising can dramatically increase the practice's goodwill. In many cases, publicity can produce a more memorable impact on public awareness than advertising.

Even though you do not control the message of a newspaper article, radio, or television story, you can have significant input into the story content. Examples of public relations include:
- Press releases of newsworthy information.
- Publicity associated with publishing articles.

Public Relations

- Publicity from involvement in civic activities.
- Publicity from radio or television appearances.
- Publicity from giving presentations to audiences in your target markets.

Press Releases

"Take calculated risks. This is quite different from being rash."
—George S. Patton

Throughout your career be aware of anything that you are doing that deserves public recognition. Send a press release to newspapers, and radio and television stations when a newsworthy event occurs. The following questions may assist you in determining if an event is newsworthy:

- Do you treat unusual diseases?
- Are you providing a new medical breakthrough technology to treat a disease?
- Are there any patients whose story is of human interest (and do you have their permission to tell it)?
- Does this story support your mission statement?

For example, most newspapers, and radio and television stations will not know that you are starting a pain management practice unless you tell them. Send a press release with pertinent information announcing that you are starting a new pain management practice. If your announcement is interesting, the news editors at the newspapers, and radio and television stations may find it newsworthy. Newsworthiness is increased if you are providing a new medical treatment that no one else in your community is providing. The following page show an example of a press release for the formation of a new practice.

FOR IMMEDIATE RELEASE

THE NEW TOWN PAIN INSTITUTE IS FOUNDED!
First Pain Management Practice to Serve the New Town Area!

New Town, Kentucky (July 6, 1999) — Drs. Jones and Smith are proud to announce the formation of The New Town Pain Institute, the first medical practice in the New Town to specialize in Pain Management, a new board certified specialty of Anesthesiology.

The New Town Pain Institute is comprised of a group of fellowship trained board certified pain management anesthesiologists who are dedicated to relieving pain disorders. The New Town Pain Institute is pleased to provide inpatient and outpatient services at the following facilities: Acme Regional Medical Center, New Town Hospital, and Lane Surgery Center.

The physicians at The New Town Pain Institute are David Jones, M.D. and Mary Smith, M.D. Both physicians are fellowship trained and board certified in Pain Management by the American Board of Anesthesiology.

Dr. David Jones received his medical degree from Mount Sinai School of Medicine. He did his residency in anesthesiology at Ohio State University and his fellowship in pain management at the Cleveland Clinic where he served as Chief Pain Fellow. His special interests include back pain and headache management.

Dr. Mary Smith received her medical degree from University of Chicago School of Medicine. She did her residency in anesthesiology and fellowship in pain management at the Cleveland Clinic. Her special interests include back pain and cancer pain management.

Both doctors treat the following pain disorders:
- Cancer Pain

Public Relations

- Headache
- Back Pain
- Head and Neck Pain
- Neuralgia (including Shingles)
- Complex Regional Pain Syndrome (formerly called Reflex Sympathetic Dystrophy)
- Causalgia
- Phantom Limb Pain
- Arthritis
- Facial Pain
- Rib Fracture Pain
- Musculoskeletal Pain

For more information about The New Town Pain Institute call (502) 555-1000
Springs Medical Plaza, 1000 Fifth Avenue, Suite 120, New Town, Kentucky 47772-4302

Published Articles

"Becoming a star may not be your destiny, but being the best that you can be is a goal that you can set for yourself."
–Bryan Lindsay

Write articles to be published in local newspapers, state or county medical society publications, medical journals, or other trade journals. Editors of magazines and professional journals are constantly looking for new material and are eager for well-written informative articles. Write an interesting article that is well-researched and directed to your target audience. Telephone the editor and state who you are and that you have written an article that would be of interested to her/his readers. Inquire about their submissions policy. If the editor in interested, send the article with a letter which "sells" the article to the editor. Follow up in a week to see if she/he is interested in publishing it. If not, send it to another publication. Be persistent. Being published, especially in quality publications, enhances creditability and fame. In addition, some publications will pay authors for articles. When your article is published, be sure to get plenty of copies from the publisher, and have re-prints printed by a professional printer on glossy paper stock. Include this in your educational package (for more information on educational package, see pages 97-99).

Civic Activities

"Nothing makes a prince so much esteemed as the undertaking of great enterprises and the setting of a noble example of his own person."
–N. Machiavelli

Participate in civic activities such as health fairs, fundraisers, or other charity events, such as the American Cancer Society Golf Tournament, the Arthritis Foundation Telethon, or March of Dimes Walkathon. If possible, get a group from your practice together in logo T-shirts to participate. In addition to providing you with a feeling of community involvement, these events give you an opportunity to meet the civic and corporate leadership of your community and promote the public relations image that you care. However, do not participate if you are not interested in these causes, because there is no publicity worse than bad publicity.

Radio and Television Appearances

"Do not try to imitate the lark of the nightingale, if you can't do it. If it's your destiny to croak like a toad, then go ahead!

Public Relations

And with all your might! Make them hear you!"
–Louis-Ferdinand Celine

Many television and radio programs have health programs that welcome physicians who have something interesting to communicate. To find out which stations have health programs, contact radio and television stations in your community. If they do have a health program, be prepared to explain your qualifications and topics that you can discuss. Then follow-up by sending a letter. Hopefully, the producer will find your topic interesting and invite you to be a guest. If you obtain a guest appearance, be sure to be professionally dressed and completely prepared. Don't participate if you are unable to articulate intelligently because no publicity is worse than bad publicity.

CHAPTER 14
Test Marketing

"Results? Why man, I have gotten a lot of results. I know 50,000 things that won't work."
–Thomas Edison

"Be willing to make decisions. That's the most important quality in a good leader. Don't fall victim to what I call the "ready-aim-aim-aim syndrome." You must be willing to fire."
–T. Boone Pickens

"Failures are like skinned knees — painful, but superficial."
–H. Ross Perot

"Good people are good because they've come to wisdom through failure. We get very little wisdom from success, you know."
–William Saroyan

Sometimes it is not always clear where you should advertise, what your message should be, or how often you should advertise. When unsure, gauge the reaction to your promotion by conducting a test. Test marketing helps determine how successful an ad campaign is by monitoring response and demand for your services as a result of a specific message or promotion (e.g. a direct mail campaign, an ad in a small local newspaper,

Test Marketing

or an ad in a directory). Using a limited budget, try different techniques and monitor the results, testing each thoroughly before investing a lot of money.

To conduct a test, select a media and a message, run an ad for a limited period of time, monitor the results, and calculate the cost per patient generated by the ad by dividing cost of the ads by the number of new patients that it generated. When conducting a test, make sure that it is the only advertising that you are doing during that period. If the promotion get results, then commit to a full-scale campaign.

Test marketing can be used to compare media such as newspapers, radio stations, cable TV, and direct mail. Test marketing can also be used to compare different messages in the same media. For example, you may find that newspaper ads in the lifestyle section get more results than ads in the health section. Or, you may learn that a certain radio program generates more patients than another. Once you know what works in your market, your practice can use the successful techniques and messages to generate results.

Test marketing is a cost-effective way to uncover flaws in your promotion. For example, assume that you want to know if newspaper ads will be effective. There are two newspapers in your community, one with a small and another with a large circulation. Both papers publish a health section on Sundays that is read by referring doctors and potential patients. The smaller paper charges $300 per ad and the larger paper charges $1000 for the same size ad.

To conduct a test, determine the message, frequency, and placement of the ad. Then create an ad that you believe will get results. Knowing that it takes at least three exposures to a message to get results, run the ad in the Sunday Health Section of the small newspaper for six consecutive weeks. When the ad is running, monitor the number of new patients who resulted directly or indirectly (if possible) from the newspaper ad. At the end of six weeks, determine the cost of generating a new patient through advertising by dividing cost of the ads by the number of new patients that it generated.

The Keys to Successful Marketing

In this example, the ads cost $1,800 ($300 per ad for six weeks) and generated 60 patients. The cost per patient is $30. If the same ad generated 100 patients, then the cost per patient is $18. Make sure the patients generated by the ads were appropriate, that is, patients who have diseases that the practice specializes in treating. An appropriate patient may be a patient with shingles, back pain, or headaches. An inappropriate patient may be a patient who has a broken arm, hearing loss, or coronary artery disease. If the ad was effective, then run it in the other newspaper for six weeks and monitor the results. Measure the cost per patient and appropriateness of patients generated by the ad in the larger newspaper. Was the cost per patient higher or lower?

If the newspaper with the larger circulation generated 150 patients in the same six-week period, then the cost per patient was $40 ($1,000 per ad for six weeks or $6,000 divided by 150 patients). Depending upon the cost per patient, you may decide to run in one, both, or neither of these papers.

It is important to also understand what an average patient is worth to the practice. For example, lets assume that the average back pain patient is seen for an initial consult (new patient office visit), three procedures, and two follow-up visits. Further, let's assume that the practice is reimbursed $75 for a new patient office visit, $275 for a lumbar epidural, and $40 for a follow-up office visit. Then the average back pain patient is worth $980. Patients' worth can be calculated by a group of all patients, or more accurately by pain disorder. To calculate the patients worth by a group, take the net income (receipts) for the practice for a given period of time (e.g. month, quarter, or year) and divide it by the number of new patients. The longer the period of time used, the more accurate the calculation. For example, if the previous years' net income from pain management was $1,200,000, and the number of patients seen was 1,400, then the average patient is worth $857.

It is also important to remember that referring doctors and potential patients may hear your message, respond positively, but not act on it because they do not have a need at the present time. When this happens, your advertising expenditures are an investment for the future. For example, let's assume that a family practice physician hears your message but currently does not have any patients who have pain disorders. But, two months later, she/he may have an appropriate patient to refer to your practice. The key to successful marketing is keeping your practice's name in mind, so that when an appropriate patient exists, you get the referral.

The Keys to Successful Marketing

CHAPTER 15
Creating an Effective Marketing Plan

"If one advances confidently in the direction of his dreams, and endeavors to live the life which he has imagined, he will meet with success unexpected in common terms."
–Henry David Thoreau

"Slow and steady wins the race."
–Aesop

An effective marketing plan is a straightforward document that defines how you are going to obtain business. The marketing plan answers the question, "How are you going to achieve the mission and goals of the practice?"

Like the strategic plan, a marketing plan is not a complex or lengthy document. It is usually three or four typewritten pages in length. The key to creating an effective marketing plan is to thoroughly analyze the practice that you want, identify how you can best obtain that practice, and follow through with what you have planned. Putting your plan in writing affirms and communicates how you are going to generate business.

Like the strategic plan, the marketing plan is not a document that is set on the shelf. Successful practices implement their plan,

Creating an Effective Marketing Plan

realizing that it takes time and frequency to reach target markets and convert them into customers. Once you create the plan, change it only for compelling reasons. It is consistency that will accomplish your goals. After the plan is developed, review it once a year, or as your environment changes, to ensure that you are still on course.

The following case study is an example of a marketing plan created for the New Town Pain Institute, a practice with two physicians. The mission of the New Town Pain Institute is:

To establish eminence in the field of pain management by providing quality, comprehensive, and cost-effective medical care by fellowship trained, board certified pain management anesthesiologists for the treatment of patients who suffer from acute, chronic, and cancer pain disorders.

The New Town Pain Institute's target markets are the following, ordered by the groups with largest number of potential referrals:

- Orthopedic Surgery
- Neurosurgery
- Neurology
- Physical Medicine and Rehabilitation
- Internal Medicine
- Family Practice
- Oncology
- Rheumatology
- Workers' Compensation Case Nurses
- Litigation Attorneys
- Insurance Carriers
- Health Care Professionals
- General Public

The New Town Pain Institute is targeting the following diseases in priority order:
- Back Pain
- Headache

The Keys to Successful Marketing

- Head and Neck Pain
- Musculoskeletal Pain
- Neuralgia (including shingles)
- Cancer
- Complex Regional Pain Syndrome (formerly called Reflex Sympathetic Dystrophy)
- Causalgia
- Phantom Limb Pain
- Arthritis
- Facial Pain
- Post-Trauma Pain
- Rib Fracture Pain
- Pain from Paraplegia or Quadriplegia

It is a goal of The New Town Pain Institute to have more than three exposures to its target markets in the first three months of practice. As you can see from the following marketing plan, they started practicing on July 1, 1999. In July, they sent out an announcement card. In August they had an open house. Then in September they mailed an introduction letter and an information kit. Their target markets received three direct mail pieces in the first three months that they were practice. In addition, their target markets will also have an opportunity to hear them speak and to see their listings in several directories and ads publications. The more frequently that the target markets hear the New Town Pain Institute's message, the more likely that they will remember them and refer patients.

Creating an Effective Marketing Plan

EXAMPLE OF A MARKETING PLAN

NEW TOWN PAIN INSTITUTE MARKETING PLAN
Business to be launched on July 1, 1999
Plan as of May 19, 1999

A. *Marketing Tools* — work with Terry Scott, a graphic artist at Creative Concepts Advertising, to develop logo and colors. The literature should incorporate the positioning statement, "Dedicated to Relieving Your Pain!" The following tools are to be developed:

1. Letterhead
2. Envelopes
3. Business cards
4. Appointment cards
5. Announcement cards with logo on outside and message on inside and corresponding envelope
6. Additional announcement cards, blank inside, to be used when sending a gift to new doctors and for thank you notes
7. Invitations to the open house and corresponding envelope
8. Paper napkins with the logo and positioning statement for the open house
9. Reminder post cards
10. Rolodex® cards
11. Brochures
12. Educational Package Folders

    Once created, obtain bids from three qualified printers. Printing must be completed by 6/01/99.

B. *Announcement Cards* will be mailed to members of the New Town County Medical Society (NTCMS), friends, family members, hospital administrators, nursing personnel, managed care company employees, and workers compensation caseworkers. Purchase a diskette containing a list of the names and addresses of the members from NTCMS. Add other names to the mailing list and create mailing labels with bar coding that have been sorted in zip code order so that the lowest bulk postage rates can be utilized. Red Postage Services will perform the mailing. The Announcement Cards are to be mailed July 1, 1999.

C. *Yellow Page Ads and Professional Directories*
1. Yellow Page Ad — The cut-off date for space commitment in the New Town Yellow Pages is 5/25/99. The art deadline is 6/15/99. The Yellow Pages will be distributed the first of November. The practice has committed to a bold listing in the Yellow Pages with no art.
2. White Page Ad — The cut-off date for space in the New Town White Pages is 8/15/99. The White Pages will be distributed in the first of January 2000. The practice has committed to a bold listing in the White Pages.
3. New Town County Medical Society — As a member of the NTCMS, there is no charge for listing both doctors with their picture and biographical information in the NTCMS directory. The forms have been completed, but still need to obtain a black and white passport size photo of each doctor. The deadline is October 15, 1999. The directory will be published in January of 2000.

Creating an Effective Marketing Plan

    4. Kentucky Medical Association —As a member of the KMA, there is no charge to be listed in this directory. The information form was completed and mailed to the KMA. The directory will be published in November of 1999.

    5. American Association of Anesthesiologists — As a member of the ASA, there is no charge to be listed in this directory. The information was completed and mailed to the ASA. The directory will be published in October of 1999.

    6. American Medical Association — As a member of the AMA, there is no charge to be listed in the directory. The information was completed and mailed to the AMA. The directory will be published in December of 1999.

D. *Professional Societies Newspapers and Magazines*

    New Town County Medical Society News — Beginning in June of 1999 and continuing for one year, the practice will be running a full-page ad in the NTCMS News magazine. At least two ads will be developed. The first ad will announce that the practice is now in business beginning July of 1999, and will run for three months (June–August). Then beginning in September, the second ad will run describing the benefits and services offered. It will run for the next nine months (September–May).

E. *Professional Vendor Booth* — a marketing display for the booth will need to be developed.

    1. New Town Association of Occupational Health Nurses (NTAOHN) annual meeting will be held on September 17-18, 1999, at the Holiday Inn South.

The Keys to Successful Marketing

      Space commitment and payment is due by August 28, 1999.
  2. New Town Cancer Nursing Association (NTCNA) annual meeting will be held on October 22-23, 1999, at the Marriott East. Space commitment and payment is due by October 1, 1999.
  3. New Town County Medical Society (NTCMS) annual meeting will be held on April 14-16, 1999, at the Hyatt Hotel in New Town. Space commitment and payment is due by March 15, 1999.

F. *Professional Speaking Engagements*
  1. Acme Regional Medical Center lecture will be "An Introduction to Pain Management", and will be given by Dr. Jones at the medical staff meeting on July 14, 1999.
  2. New Town Hospital lecture will be "An Introduction to Pain Management", and will be given by Dr. Jones at the medical staff meeting on August 4, 1999.
  3. Lane Surgery Center lecture will be "An Introduction to Pain Management", and will be given by Dr. Smith at the medical staff meeting on August 20, 1999.
  4. New Town Hospital Health and Information Center lecture will be "An Introduction to Pain Management", and will be given by Dr. Smith to the general public on September 12, 1999.
  5. New Town Hospital Health and Information Center lecture will be "Back Pain – You Don't Have to Live in Pain", and will be given by Dr. Smith to the general public on November 14, 1999.
  6. New Town Workers Compensation Insurance Company lecture will be "Pain Management: A Cost Effective Approach to Treating Pain", and

Creating an Effective Marketing Plan

will be given by Dr. Smith to nurses employed as a caseworker at the staff meeting on November 20, 1999.

7. New Town Hospital Health and Information Center lecture will be "An Introduction to Pain Management", and will be given by Dr. Jones to the general public on January 23, 2000.

G. *Open House* will be held on August 6, 1999, from 4:00 p.m. until 7:00 p.m. at the office. Complete hors d'oeuvres will be served as well as champagne, wine, beer and soft drinks.

H. *Public Relations* — A press release announcing that the Institute is the first pain center in New Town will be sent to the following:

1. *New Town Star Newspaper*
2. *New Town County Medical Society Magazine*
3. Acme Regional Medical Center Newsletter
4. New Town Hospital Newsletter
5. Lane Surgery Center Newsletter
6. TV Channel 3 Health Watch
7. TV Channel 5 Medical Update
8. TV Channel 9 local news
9. AM radio stations: 77.2 and 80.6
10. FM radio stations: 98.7, 101.4, and 107.42.

I. *Promotional Items*
   1. Coffee Cups
   2. Pens

J. *Plant for New Doctors* — A peace lily potted plant filled with fresh flowers will be sent to

145

The Keys to Successful Marketing

every new doctor in the target markets. The card will have our logo on the outside and the inside will contain a handwritten note stating: "Wishing you success." Both physicians will sign the card.

K. *The Doctors Lounge* – It is the goal of the practice that the physicians will stop by doctors' lounges and meet potential referring doctors.

L. *Potential Referring Doctor Office Visits* – Practices have been divided into two groups. The first group includes Orthopedic Surgery, Neurosurgery, and Neurology to whom lunch will be taken. The second group includes Physical Medicine and Rehabilitation, Internal Medicine, Family Practice, Oncology, and Rheumatology to whom bagels, muffins, and cream cheese will be taken. Within each group, the number of doctors and the likelihood for referring patients will be used to prioritize the order in which the referring doctor practices will be called upon. The following items will also be given to the physicians and their staff:

1. Educational package folder
2. Introduction letter
3. Brochure
4. Business card
5. Rolodex® card
6. Coffee cup
7. Pens

M. *Seasons Greetings* — On or about December 1, 1999, a seasons' greetings card will be mailed to all referring doctors, friends, family members, hospital administrators, nursing personnel, managed care company employees, and workers' compensation caseworkers

N. *Insurance Participation* — It will be a goal of the practice to participate with most managed care companies. The practice will not participate with managed care companies whose reimbursement is so low that it is not economically feasible.

O. *Direct Mail* — In September of 1999, an introduction letter, brochure, Rolodex® card, and business card will be mailed to the members of the New Town County Medical Society, hospital administrators, nursing personnel, managed care company employees, and workers' compensation caseworkers.

P. *Newspaper Ads* will be placed four times during the year, once in each of the Health Care Quarterly special sections of the *New Town Star Newspaper*.

Q. *Radio* — On August 8, 1999, Dr. Jones will answer questions on back pain as a guest speaker on "Health Talk", a radio program on 80.6 AM.

R. *Publish Articles* — It is a goal of the practice to write two articles on pain management topics and have them published by May of 2000.

S. *Quality Improvement* — Both a patient satisfaction survey and a referring doctor survey will be created and utilized.
   1. Patient Satisfaction Survey — At the conclusion of his or her appointment, each patient will be given a patient satisfaction survey. Suggestions will be used to improve the

quality of services rendered. A commitment has been made to have sufficient personnel to telephone patients who ask to speak to someone about their service.

2. Referring Doctor Survey — In February of 2000, all physicians who have referred at least one patient to the practice will be mailed a referring doctor satisfaction survey. Suggestions will be used to improve the quality of the services rendered. The physicians have committed to telephoning referring doctors who ask to speak to someone about their service.

CARPE DIEM
(LATIN: SEIZE THE DAY)

–HORACE

Postscript

The author, Linda M. Van Horn, M.B.A., is writing several more books on pain management topics. Her next book is entitled, *Building a Successful Pain Management Practice: The Keys to Establishing and Running an Efficient Practice*. This book contains information on the business tools needed for start-up, the contents of a medical and billing chart, facility planning, staffing, telephone skills, and scheduling. To find out more information or to get your name on the mailing list for the next book, please call or write 21st Century Edge at:

21st Century Edge, Inc.

1701 Spruce Lane

Louisville, Kentucky 40207

(502) 721-9170

(877) 214-EDGE

References

1. Barnett M.D., Albert E. and Mayer R.N., EdD, FAAN, Gloria Gilbert. *Ambulatory Care Management and Practice.* Gaithersburg, Maryland: An Aspen Publication, 1992.

2. Eliscu, Andrea. *Position for Success! Strategic Marketing for Group Practices.* Englewood, Colorado: Medical Group Management Association, 1995.

3. Freeman, Edward R. *Strategic Management: A Stakeholder Approach.* Marchfiled, Massachusetts: Pitman Publishing Inc., 1984.

4. Kazmier, Leonard. *Statistical Analysis for Business and Economics.* New York, New York: McGraw-Hill Book Company, 1978.

5. Kotler, Philip, Ph.D. *Marketing Management Analysis, Planning and Cost Control 4th Edition.* Englewood Cliffs, New Jersey: Prentice-Hall, Inc., 1980.

6. Kotler, Philip, Ph.D. *Principles of Marketing.* Englewood Cliffs, New Jersey: Prentice-Hall, Inc., 1980.

7. Korenchuck, J.D., M.P.H. Keith. *Transforming the Delivery of Health Care: Mergers, Acquisitions and Physician-Hospital Organizations.* Englewood, Colorado: Medical Group Management Association, 1992.

8. Lesikar, Raymond, V. *Business Communication Theory and Application 4th Edition.* Homewood, Illinois: Richard D. Irwin, Inc., 1980.

9. Levin, Richard L. and Kirkpatrick, Charles, A. *Quantitative Approaches to Management 4th Edition.* New York, New York: McGraw-Hill Book Company, 1978.

10. Peppers, Don and Rogers, Ph.D., Martha. *The One to One Future: Building Relationships One Customer at a Time.* New York, New York: DoubleDay, 1993.

11. Ross, M.P.H., Austin, Schafer P.A., and Williams, Sc.D., Stephen. *Ambulatory Care Management 2nd Edition.* Albany, New York: Delmar Publishers, Inc., 1991.

12. Slaton, Ed.D., FACMPE, Robert, Manning, Bob, and Jack-

References

son, Clyde. *From Green Persimmons to Cranky Parrots: Practice Management Axioms to Live By*. Englewood, Colorado: Medical Group Management Association, 1993.

13. Stoner, James A.F. *Management*. Englewood Cliffs, New Jersey: Prentice-Hall Inc., 1978.

14. Strickland, III., A.J., and Thompson, Jr., Arthur A. *Cases in Strategic Management*. Plano, Texas: Business Publication, Inc., 1982.

15. Strickland, III., A.J., and Thompson, Jr., Arthur A. *Strategy and Policy: Concepts and Cases*. Plano, Texas: Business Publication, Inc., 1981.

16. Strickland, III., A.J., and Thompson, Jr., Arthur A. *Strategy Formulation and Implementation: Tasks of the General Manager*. Plano, Texas: Business Publication, Inc., 1983.

17. Sullivan, Kevin and Luallin, Meryl. *The Medical Marketer's Guide Success Strategies for Group Practice Management 2nd Edition*. Englewood, Colorado, Medical Group Management Association, 1992.

18. Winwood, Richard I. *Time Management: An Introduction to the Franklin System*. Salt Lake City, Utah: Franklin International Institute, Inc., 1990.

19. ———. *1998 Relative Value Guide: A Guide for Anesthesia Value*. Park Ridge, Illinois: American Society of Anesthesiologists, 1998

20. ———. *Physician Fee Analyzer Plus*. Salt Lake City, Utah: Medicode, 1996.

21. ———. *Writing an Effective Business Plan*, New York, New York: Deloitte & Touche.

INDEX

Advertising and Selling, 80-82
Advertising media, *see* media 120-127
Announcement, 87-89
    Illustration of, 88-89
Appointment card, 90-91
    Illustration of, 91
Business Card, 90
    Illustration of, 90
Brochures, 94-96
    Illustration of, 95-96
Civic activities, *see* public relations
Competitive analysis, 22-23
    Questions to assist in definition of, 22-23
Direct mail, 101-103
Directories, 103-105
Doctors lounge, 112
Educational packages, 97-99
Ethics in Patients Referrals Act (Stark Legislation), 116-119
Federal Anti-Kickback Statute, 115-116
Fee schedule, *see* pricing
Goodwill, 70-74
    Definition of, 70
    Increasing, 101, 105-107, 109, 121, 128

Index

Goals of the practice, 28-30
   Example of, 29-30
   Measurement of, 29-30
   Time Frame, 29
   Subject, 28
Introduction letters, 97
   Illustration of, 98
Legal Entities, 75-79
   C Corporation, 76-78
   Example of Sub-chapter S set-up, 79
   Limited Liability Company, 79
   Limited Liability Partnership, 76
   Non-profit Organization, 78-79
   Partnership, 76
   Sole Proprietorship, 75
   Sub-Chapter S Corporation, 78
Logo, 72-73
Marketing office visits, 112-114
Marketing plan, 138-148
   Example of, 141-148
Market research, 36-46
   Complaint, 39
   Example of patient satisfaction survey, 41-43
   Example of referring doctor satisfaction survey, 44-46
   Satisfaction surveys, 38-40
Marketing, 31-148
   Definition of, 32
   Goal of, 32
Media, 120-127
   Billboards, 123
   Internet, 126-127
   Magazines, 123-124
   Newspapers and newsletters, 122-123

Index

Radio, 124-125
Television (regular and cable), 125-126
Mission statement, 13-15
    Definition of, 13
    Examples of, 14-15
    Questions to assist in definition of, 14
Naming the practice, 71-72
Need, 33-34
    Definition of, 33
    Example of, 34
    Services to satisfy, *see* service development
Needs assessment, 33-35
Newsletters, 100
New physicians, 110-111
Occasional correspondence, 119
Office visits, *see* marketing office visits
Outgoing referrals, 115-119
Position statement, 73-74
Presentations to target markets, 108-110
Press release, *see* public relations
Pricing, 53-69
    Analyze the data, 58-69
    ASA Relative Value, 57-58
    ASA Relative Value Method, 59-62
    Cost Plus Pricing Method, 62-64
    Figure 1: ASA Relative Value Method, 60-61
    Figure 2: Cost Plus Pricing Method, 63-64
    Figure 3: Marketplace Average Method, 66-67
    Figure 4: Analysis of All Methods, 68-69
    Finalize fee schedule, 64-65
    Identify every procedure, 54
    Marketplace Average Method, 64
    Medicare Part B fee schedule, 54-57

Index

    Reimbursement Information, 58
    Steps to create a fee schedule, 53
Professional societies, 107-108
Promotional items, 105-107
Public relations, 128-133
    Civic activities, 132
    Illustration of press release, 130-131
    Press release, 129-131
    Published Articles, 131-132
    Radio and television appearances, 132-133
Published articles, *see* public relations
Radio and television appearances, *see* public relations
Reminder postcards, 91-93
    Illustration of computer generated, 92
    Illustration of hand written, 93
Rollodex® Cards, 94
    Illustration of, 94
Satisfaction Survey, *see* market research
Seasonal Correspondence, 119
Service Development, 49-52
    Example of services, 50-52
Servicemark, 74
Stark Legislation, *see* Ethics in Patients Referrals Act
Strategy formation, 10
Strategic Planing, 10-30
    Contents of, 11-12
    Purpose of, 10-11
SWOT, 24-27
    Definition of, 24
    Questions to assist in definition of opportunities, 26
    Questions to assist in definition of strengths, 25
    Questions to assist in definition of threats, 27
    Questions to assist in definition of weakness, 26

Target markets, 16-21
    Advertising to, *see* advertising and selling
    Assessing practice to determine needs and wants, 37-38
    Questions to assist in definition of, 18-19
    Needs and wants of, 33-35
    Satisfaction of needs and wants, 32, 47-48
    Satisfaction surveys, *see* market research
    Services for, *see* service development
    Sources for demographic information on, 20-21
Test marketing, 134-137
Timing and packaging, 83-85
Trademark, 74
Want, 33-34
    Creation of, 47-48
    Definition of, 34
    Services to satisfy, *see* service development